How to Seduce Your Dream Man

100 strategies to bring Mr Right to heel

how to

SEDUCE
YOUR DREAM
MAN

100 strategies to bring Mr Right to heel

ANNA MAXTED

Thorsons
An Imprint of HarperCollins*Publishers*

Thorsons
An Imprint of HarperCollins*Publishers*
77–85 Fulham Palace Road,
Hammersmith, London W6 8JB

The Thorsons website address is:
www.thorsons.com

Published by Thorsons in association with
Cosmopolitan magazine and Hearst Communications, Inc., 1999
Cosmopolitan is a trademark of
Hearst Communications, Inc.

1 3 5 7 9 10 8 6 4 2

Anna Maxted asserts the moral right to
be identified as the author of this work

A catalogue record for this book
is available from the British Library

ISBN 0 7225 3901 0

Printed and bound in Great Britain by
Caledonian International Book Manufacturing Ltd, Glasgow

To Phil Robinson

Contents

STAGE 3: *First Organized Date*   115

Introduction

Finding your Dream Man can be more tedious, dispiriting and frustrating than public transport on a leafy day. Where the hell is he? Is he going to take 37 years to arrive? Did you miss him by four seconds because you had a third slice of toast? Stop flapping. The wonderful thing about the Dream Man is, he wants to find you too. The hallowed myth about men fainting at the word commitment (woo! creepy!) is hollow myth. Men do want to commit – to the right woman – and are only scared of being ridiculed by their stormingly jealous single friends. All of whom rely heavily on the pizza delivery boy as their main source of human contact and who haven't had sex with anyone bar their own right hand for eighteen months.

The infuriating thing about the average Dream Man, however, is he often avoids you for years. Worse, when you finally sashay into his line of blue-eyed vision the goon doesn't glance up from his pint. You are reduced to wondering, would you have more success if you exchanged your little black dress for a hops barrel? Enough wondering. Your Dream Man is within reach, and together we'll nail him (in the nicest possible way, of course.) We will also have enormous fun finding him. We are going to travel first class, which means you don't have to tromp from bar to bar to bar day in day out, feet raw from tromping, eyes peeled from searching.

Once you've brought Mr Right to heel – and there are a wealth of strategies to lure him there so take your pick – the next trick is getting him to sit and stay. Not a problem. These seductive techniques are easy to master – and so is he. All you require is a little front. Cats do this by fluffing up their tails to make themselves look bigger and more impressive than they really are. Well as if that fools anyone. We will do it by wile and guile, judicious make-up, and the knowledge that if he takes the bait it will be the best thing that ever happened to him. Believe it, go for it, and get him. Then, of course – so long as he does his fair share of the washing up – all will be pink and fluffy for ever.

Pre-Man Preparation

Positive thinking empowers you, as does a nice pair of boots. We shall employ every ruse possible to ensure that when your eyes finally meet, yours smoulder sexily while his practically pop from their sockets. Begin here...

Believing You're It

This doesn't mean swaggering around like the school bully boasting about your achievements, it means retaining an inner conviction of your own attractiveness and worth. This lends a glow to a woman and – trite as it sounds – it truly is the most important part of nabbing Mr Right. Self-confidence is seductive. It convinces men (and women) you have something to feel confident about. If you believe you're special, everyone wants a piece of you. Which piece they get is up to you.

Whereas if, when you meet a potential candidate for life partnership, you say things like 'I think such and such but then, what do I know?' that self-denigration will rub off on him. If you persist in saying 'I'm rubbish at relation-ships' and 'I'm such a frump' he may start to believe you. Think of yourself as your own PR woman. You have to sell yourself and the most convincing way you can do it is to believe your own hype. That means being nice to and about yourself. So:

A) Quit the false modesty. Men don't go in for it so they don't really understand it. They'll offer reassurance to be polite, but they won't admire you for it.

B) Don't ever draw attention to your worst features in a beat-them-to-it mindset. Saying 'I've got a profile like a witch – my nose and chin practically meet!' – when, in fact both features are just ever so slightly curved – only draws his attention to an until now unperceived imperfection. Now that's berkish.

C) If he makes a reference to something and you haven't the least idea what it is don't fall into a panicky negative state of mind – 'I'm so stupid, now he's going to think I'm a dunce', etc. If you suspect it is kindergarten general knowledge which has inexplicably passed you by, bluff. If he asks your opinion say, 'I can't really make up my mind about this, what do you think?' Then, as soon as you can, change the subject. If however, he's gabbing about his pet subject there is no shame in saying brightly 'Sorry, but I don't know what that is.' Note, you don't have to preface your admission with useless self-flagellating nonsense like, 'I must be really thick but … ' A straightforward admission is refreshingly blunt and if he's Mr Right material he'll appreciate that. Also, men love explaining.

Clothes to Make Him Dribble

The idea being to look jaw-droppingly sexy without seeming to tout for business. This means balance and subtlety. If you know you look ravishing in boots and hotpants, you don't need to wear a low-cut top as well. The majority of men – in their great wisdom and conceit – will assume you're gagging for it. This may have them clustering around you like dogs around a chocolate biscuit, but at the same time it robs you of power. You want them to be gagging for it, and to be wondering, hoping, possibly, if they're really good, might they maybe have a chance with you?

The way to confuse them is to wear one devastatingly raunchy item – or, at least, an item with devastatingly raunchy effect – and cover up the rest. This way, they are more respectful, less cocky. You also weed out the bumptious bores who think that if a woman doesn't dress like Pauline Calf she must be a lesbian. Here's how to tantalize the rest of them. Starting with the basics:

- The nipple outline: men are riveted by nipples. Their attention cannot be swayed. While a perky cleavage also does the trick, it also suggests – in his sexist head – that you're up for it. Better that he thinks he's persuading you to be up for it. This way you are a challenge. Men think they want an easy lay because they are lazy and easily influenced by their loutish friends. But, if they feel you have been too compliant (don't torture yourself with the hypocrisy, it's not worth it) they are less likely to appreciate you for the gorgeous, they-should-be-so-lucky creature you are. It's ridiculous, it's tedious, it's a waste of everyone's time, but a man loves to feel he's had to chase a woman. Even though his mother buys his clothes for him and he lives on takeaways, he thinks of himself as a hunter. Which means that, unlike a cavernous cleavage, a nipple outline through a thin t-shirt and bra (and feel free to go to the ladies and pinch them till they stand to attention) will focus his gaze without him thinking he's being manipulated. As if.

■ Off-the shoulder top: it makes him realize that very possibly you are not wearing a bra. Men can weave a three-hour fantasy on that basic premise. They gawk, they wonder, they approach. If your bosom droops without support, however, go to the other extreme — hoick everything up and together. You don't have to look like an Elizabethan serving wench; a slight bulge is enough to tantalize. Again, if you're making the most of your chest, don't wear peel-off trousers.

■ No knickers: best if you're wearing a long skirt. The idea is not to flash your bits like a baboon, but let him puzzle over the absence of knickerline, wonder 'Can she be wearing underwear?' Gets him hot under the boxers.

- Knee-high boots and — if you really want to give him a kick — jodhpurs. Frankly, jodhpurs make anyone's hips look a mile wide but men love clothes that emphasize a woman's curves and encourage them to imagine her with a riding crop in her hand. A tip — lose the riding hat.

- Zip up top: he can't tear his mind away from the idea of grabbing the zip and pulling...

- White, slightly sheer shirt with the two top buttons undone — enough to afford him a glimpse of bra, preferably white, lacy. If you want bigger bosoms invest in a padded bra. Most men wouldn't know a padded bra if it bit them, so don't worry about him thinking you're faking.

- Skirt with a small slit in it. (He thinks wow, her legs go all the way up ...)

- Non-flat shoes. Flat shoes are so dowdy, unless they're state of the art trainers there's no excuse for them. Even Malono Blahniks, even the most designery, showy-offy, straight from the catwalk flat shoes cut no ice with men, unless they work in fashion or retail and can recognize and shallowly appreciate them for the style statement they are. Otherwise, most men are suckers for a woman in heels. They make your legs look endless, even if you're 5 feet 2 inches, and they add a wiggle to your walk. They don't have to be crippling either — and when you're man hunting it's best to wear your reliable heels rather than your spangly untried new ones, or halfway through the evening you'll find yourself walking like a hobgoblin.*

---

* If you ignore this advice, wear your spikiest, highest, most lethal dagger heels and as he offers to walk you home, feel as though you may faint from pain, the sexiest thing you can do is to take off your shoes and walk barefoot. Subtext: hey! wild, free-spirited me! I'm not bound by convention! (Only look out for dog poo on the pavement or your fey but cute pose will be shot to smithereens.)

Wedding or Funeral Attire?

All the sages say don't wear black as men don't like black, apparently. It's true that you rarely see men themselves wearing black, and if they are, they're usually wannabees in the music business. However, if you think you look delectable in black, Mr Right will think the same. Truth is, the kind of men who don't like women wearing black are their fathers and elderly male relatives, the sort who say, when you were under the impression you were looking rather fit, 'My dear, you look so sombre – you need to wear some nice jolly colours and put on a bit of weight. Mavis! Another helping of macaroni cheese for my favourite niece! And Mavis! That orange and purple jumper you were knitting for your sister-in-law, I think madam here needs it!'

Younger men are suckers for a woman who dresses judiciously in black. Which means if she does look like she's going to a funeral, it's a damn slinky one. Women with dark hair tend to look ravishing in black. Black is flattering, sophisticated, and black trousers with black boots make your legs look longer than they really are. If you're happy to make a concession and wear something non-black, make it your top (depending of course on whether you want to maximize or minimize). The little black dress is only a cliché because it's practically infallible.

Making Him Think You're a Natural Beauty

This requires a ton of work. The joyous thing is, you can slap on piles of carefully, delicately applied make-up, and he will think you're wearing nothing but the glorious features God gave you. This is our goal. What is not, is for you to paste it on as if you were plastering a ceiling. Men don't like women who wear too much make-up. Make-up that, if it fell off, would crack the pavement. It reminds them of scary old ladies bending down to engulf them in a perfume-reeky kiss when they were aged five. It suggests you have something to hide. Make-up is not to disguise (apart from the odd blemish and uneven skin tone) it is to enhance. If you are under 55, you do not need heaps of make-up. If you look too powdery he'll think 'Urk, I could scrape my finger down that and leave a hollow'.

Counter make-up artists are the worst offenders – they have products to sell and so want to use every one of them. They try to convince you that to survive ridicule you need to look like Pinocchio. Whereas, in the real world your man does not want to think that if he kisses you your face will come off on him. So – easy on the foundation – and concentrate on enhancing your features. Which you can do by the following:

- Have plucked eyebrows, not over-plucked. Pluck stray hairs from underneath the brow, and if you're not a natural eyebrow plucker, go to a beautician – with a picture of your ideal brow shape, so she doesn't do anything scary involving initiative.

- Bleach, or (if you're a martyr) have electrolysis to remove facial hair. Admittedly, men have got a nerve, what with their fancy goatees, and elaborate sideburns, but they are outrageously squeamish about women who have even a whisker of whiskers and call them horrid names like Van Cleef.

- Once you have the basics – neat eyebrows, no moustache – you're ready to glam up. Cleanse, moisturize (is it just me or is toning a waste of time?) then apply, preferably with clean fingertips, a veneer of liquid foundation. Don't go mad. Unless you want to look like Wurzel Gummidge's Aunt Sally you only need a little to even out your skin tone. You should still be able to see your skin. Then dust lightly with a smidge of powder just to take off the shine, not to cake. The most irritating habit faces have is to turn shiny a few hours after being made up. To combat this try a matting product, such as Estee Lauder T-Controle, or the Body Shop Papier Poudre, which blots up excess oil – fast, easy, effective.

- Use an eyelash curler (provokes compliments from men such as 'You've got lovely bendy eyelashes') and lashings of mascara to make your lashes battable. To make your eyes seem huge, apply eyeliner starting from about one-third of the way along your top lid, and two-thirds of the way along your bottom lid. Don't join up the two lines – leave approximately two millimetres between them (think Cleopatra on a quiet day). This makes your eyes look wider.
- As for your lips, the worst thing you can do if you have thin lips is apply lip liner outside them to make them look bigger. It doesn't fool anyone and it makes you look daft. The best thing to do is to avoid dark lipsticks. Incidentally, whatever your lip size, your lip liner should be the same shade as your lipstick – anything else is naff. When you apply your lipstick, blot then apply again. It's not classy to take a sip of your drink and leave a gob-shaped scarlet mark on the rim.

Note

A cute touchy-feely excuse to stroke his face on date two is to kiss him hello on the cheek, then sweetly rub off the kiss-mark with your fingers. Especially arousing for men because in some perverted way it reminds them of their mother cleaning their face when they were little. Ah!

If you feel naked without blusher, dab a little in the apples of your cheeks, but don't streak it on – two red go-faster stripes across your face will make you look like Adam Ant's sister or a souped-up Ford Escort.

Knock-Him-Out Appearance Tips

- Make sure your hair isn't flat at the back. If you haven't got time to wash it, use a dry shampoo to puff it up a bit.
- Check your teeth for green bits (carry floss in your bag) and ensure your breath is more minty than a vat of Polos, because there's nothing more off-putting than a blast of death-breath. If you haven't had a chance to brush your teeth, chew gum. But make it habit to carry a toothbrush and toothpaste – even if you can't find a sink to spit in, it won't kill you to swallow.
- Check your nose for bogies, ears for wax, hair for dandruff, eyes for sleep – basically any side-effect of being human – and exterminate.
- Clean your fingernails – nice if they're longish but not too long – when they start to go curly you know it's time to file, and moisturize your hands so they're not as rough to the touch as a rhino's elbow.
- If you wear glasses, clean them so you're not peering through smears – oh, and make sure your glasses are sexy to the point where he's dying to remove them and whisper, 'Why, but Miss Smith … you're bee-ooot-iful!'

- Use perfume in moderation — and grown up sex kittens use real perfume not sickly sweet Essence of Blackberry or anything akin to it. Whatever you choose, don't drench yourself in it like some fearsome elderly aunt. A moderate dab of good perfume will leave a whisper of scent about him, so that when you part he'll gradually become aware he can smell something gorgeous, different — wow, not eau de Silk Cut — but a delicious sexy aroma — essence of you. It's a brilliant ruse!

Showing Off Curves

Men like what they haven't got (a lesson to us all) and what they haven't got are curves. Beer bellies don't count. The way, therefore, to make them gawk is to draw their attention to your curves, and for once, we're not talking about bosoms. We can thank psychologist Devendra Singh for this theory: his research at the University of Texas in Austin showed that women, men thought of as sexy, had one thing in common – whether they were as skinny as Twiggy or as voluptuous as Marilyn Monroe – they had similarly proportionate curves, their waists being between two-thirds or 80% of the size of their hip measurement. The magnet to men therefore is not how skinny you are, it is how curvy you are. So whether you're a size 16 or a size eight, flaunt your curves. Whether you choose to do this by wearing hipsters and piercing your belly button, or by tucking your white shirt into your black skirt is up to you. Don't flap if you are a straight-down sort of shape – it's highly unlikely that your waist is larger than your hip size. You surely have some curve – emphasize it.

Self-Awareness: Tailoring Yourself to Perfection

Know what impression you give. It's probably not quite the same as you think.

Real Life, Real Wires Crossed

Tara, 27: 'I'm not very confident but I think of myself as a friendly person. If I feel comfortable I chat away, but the second I suspect the person I'm talking to isn't captivated, the facade falls away and I stammer and talk nonsense. Recently though, I felt as if I was becoming a social pariah. Although I am successful in my career, when I met up with acquaintances in the same profession I'd feel certain they were regarding me with disdain. I mentioned this to a close friend and she said "Tara, you're a very glamorous woman – but in all honesty you come across as superior and unapproachable. People are in awe of you". I could barely believe it. I think I was so nervous, I wouldn't smile in case someone didn't smile back. I had no idea. Now, I try not to grimace, and to make eye contact. It's made all the difference.'

Anyone accustomed to public speaking knows that what you say is only a tiny part of making a good impression. Your audience judges you on your expression, tone, body language, gestures, appearance. In other words, you don't need to burble all night to make him fall for you.

Tape yourself talking and, painful as it is, play it back. If you sound like a sheep calling to its young or a hysterical mouse, train yourself to slow down – this will make your voice less bleaty and/or squeaky. Count the number of times you say 'you know' or 'like' and try to eliminate what you hate about the way you express yourself. If you love every bit of it, hooray for you.

Watch yourself. If you have a habit of say, winking, check in the mirror to ensure you don't make a face like a gargoyle. If your speciality is a Jim Carey style cheesy grin, ditto.

Reassessing What You Want

Apologies — it sounds like something your mother would say. But it's a great exercise because it makes you consider exactly what you want from a relationship — rather than what you merely think you want — and it works.

How To
Make a list of all your ah, abortive relationships. Beside the name of each man (if you can remember their names) write down what traits attracted you. In the next column, note down what went wrong. In the next, what was missing from the relationship. In the next, an honest judgement of the reasons. It doesn't matter if you repeat yourself — sometimes asking the same question in slightly different forms is the best way of establishing the truth. See if any patterns emerge. Belinda, 31, who is currently engaged, kissed many a warty toad before finding her dream man. In hindsight, she can see her mistakes — and the motivation for them:

Name	Stuart
attraction	good-looking, sheepish, part of a cool crowd, laddish, different background to me.
what went wrong	he seemed to get bored, just stopped calling.
what was missing	depth, real connection.
why?	we didn't have that much in common beyond the initial attraction, too much into his laddish lifestyle to want a serious relationship, I was never part of his crowd.
Belinda's mistake	maybe I didn't want to see him as he really was. I was shocked when he went off me.

Name	Andrew
attraction	sexy, aloof, very posh (different to me), conservative, amused by me, just split with long term girlfriend.
what went wrong	we argued – about politics, the role of women, everything. He cheated on me with his ex.
what was missing	he saw me as an amusement, not as me, so I adapted my real personality.

why?	beyond the sex we had zero in common – he was a snob, repressed, he demoralized me.
Belinda's mistake	thinking I could have a relationship with someone who was aloof – I crave affection, and foolishly, the more he retreated the more I tried to wheedle it out of him. Not having the pride or self-respect to walk away.

Name	Mike
attraction	cute.
what went wrong	I got bored, he got too serious
what was missing	any real interest in him as a person, or respect for him.
why?	he was boring, had nothing to say, he irritated me – his clinginess irritated me.
Belinda's mistake	choosing looks over personality.

Name	Robert
attraction	Irish Catholic, like me.
what went wrong	I didn't fancy him enough, we had our background in common but it was almost too familiar, he was too right-on for me.
what was missing	chemistry.

why?	he was sweet, nice, but it bored me – it was like going out with your brother.
Belinda's mistake	going out with someone I didn't really fancy.
Name	Paul
attraction	cool job, amazingly good-looking, laddish, slightly little boy lost.
what went wrong	emotionally immature, rude to my friends, selfish, I stopped respecting him, I felt like his mother.
what was missing	any real respect, real compatibility, equality.
why?	he was rubbish at sex, even though I fancied him madly, and his immaturity was frustrating – it made me realize he was too young. I resented him.
Belinda's mistake	thinking that a guy so into being a lad, who was still rebelling against his parents, would be a suitable partner for me.
Mr Right	Martin
attraction	hysterically funny, intelligent, mischievous, we have great conversations, brilliant in bed,

How to Seduce Your Dream Man

laddish but also mature, very kind and not just to me, cool job, different background but a lot in common – and he is knowledgeable and respectful of my background.

any doubts

he was keen on me from the start, which put me off him. Not my usual type – not posh, no emotional problems, no game playing. Good-looking but not lust at first sight for me.

Belinda's conclusion: 'I was a fat, insecure teenager, and for many years I still thought of myself with disgust. I think that was partly why I'd go for men who were wildly different from me, which meant we had nothing in common. I'd also go for emotionally remote men – maybe I thought I didn't deserve love, but it made me miserable when I didn't get it. And the men who were keen on me like Robert and Mike, I almost despised them for it. I mostly went for looks over personality and I didn't truly respect them as people. It was different with Martin. His personality hooked me. He also makes me feel very loved and great about myself. I am never bored or uncomfortable in his company. I respect him.'

After the Assessment

According to the conclusions you reach – and it may be a good idea to ask a trustworthy friend to judge as well – give a man a chance who isn't your normal type, because if you're reading this book it may possibly be that your normal type is the wrong type for you. Some experts suggest this is because you are secretly afraid of commitment so you go for men who you know will eventually reject you, and then you can blame it not working out on them. Consider it. If you reckon this theory doesn't apply to you, we'll press on. Give the guy you were hum-ha'ing about because he didn't fit your normal criteria a chance. If you want it to be a small chance, make the date a coffee. If the date turns out to be hellish, you can suddenly produce a meeting with your sister in half an hour's time 'So I'd better leave in ten minutes.' Don't say this as you greet him, because if the date goes stormingly you will have to cut it unnecessarily short.

Learn to Ignore Toxic Attitudes

Such as friends who say things like 'all men are shits'.

Correct Answer " "
Think: Well, dating a man who refers to women as 'rides', drinks thirteen pints on a quiet night, and thinks baths are for wusses is bound to colour your judgement. Fortunately, I have better taste than you.

Peptalk
Don't let miseryguts drag you down. People who say things like this are anathema to securing Mr Right because they clog your head full of negative thoughts. If you go out thinking that all men are shits (which isn't true, it's an understatement, joke, sorry) you will not be giving out appropriate vibes. It's very easy to be whipped into a self-pitying rant against all men, and certainly, we've all indulged in it and thoroughly enjoyed ourselves. But some women take it too seriously and use it as an excuse for eating a whole packet of biscuits in one sitting. Eat the biscuits for heaven's sake – just own up to having a sweet tooth.

The 'all men are shits' attitude is not only juvenile, it is bad for your health. It's the victim mentality – 'Poor me, it's all their fault!' No doubt if miseryguts friend wasn't such a whinging bore she'd get a few more offers. Don't go out with friends like these if you're hoping to stumble across Mr Right because they'll lurk around looking about as jolly as Dracula's shadow and their Keep Off aura will scare away any potential. Not to be mean, but it's not in her interest that you score with a dream man who proves to be sexy, faithful, funny, intelligent, successful, amazing et cetera – it would put her theory out of kilter and her nose out of joint.

Dealing with Annoying Elderly Relatives

Who say 'What, no young man?' (Implication: there's something wrong with you.)

Correct answer (sweet, smiling)
'No, just one night stands.'

If you tromp away thinking 'Maybe Uncle Dicky is right, maybe I am over the hill, an oddity at 24, because I am not spending my Sundays wheeling a great trolley full of cheap tat around a stuffy home store with my devoted man and a diamond on my finger big enough to poke someone's eye out,' you will acquire an air of wild desperation. Remember that when Uncle Dicky was a lad, ladies were considered spinsters if they weren't married by the age of 17. Times have changed since the Victorian era, you might like to inform him.

Men who are Patently Not Mr Right

Any who badger you all evening and say things like 'Why isn't a nice girl like you going out with someone?' (Implication: there's something wrong with you.)

Correct Answer
'I haven't met anyone I like,' (pause, plus cool stare) 'I still haven't'.

Get away from these timewasters as fast as possible. While they yabber away, butt in mid-flow with the words, 'Excuse me' (mouth this next bit so he can't be sure what you're saying) 'you're really boring me'. Smile and walk off.

Making Contact
The scariest bit, allegedly. The pomp and puffery that surrounds the idea of men and women who don't know each other meeting in a public place for the first time, acknowledging each other and (gasp!) striking up a conversation, is bizarre. On the pull ... cattle market ... getting picked up ... Yes, and? It's natural! We'd be extinct otherwise! What

possible gripe can anyone have about someone wanting to find The One? Thanks to all the hype, searching for Mr Right can chill you with fear. In fact, it's a blast. You have much more fun than most married people. Prepare to dazzle.

Making Contact

The scariest bit, allegedly. The pomp and puffery that surrounds the idea of men and women who don't know each other meeting in a public place for the first time, acknowledging each other and (gasp!) striking up a conversation, is bizarre. On the pull … cattle market … getting picked up … Yes, and? It's natural! We'd be extinct otherwise! What possible gripe can anyone have about someone wanting to find The One? Thanks to all the hype, searching for Mr Right can chill you with fear. In fact, it's a blast. You have much more fun than most married people. Prepare to dazzle.

Flirt for Flirting's Sake

The important thing to know about flirting is that it doesn't have to have a goal. It does not have to be blatantly sexual. Flirting is a playful attitude and is a way of getting along with people. You do not have to restrict your flirtatiousness to men. You can flirt with everyone. You should. Flirtation is natural. It is instinct. You can make people swivel by squawking and moaning and behaving badly. Or by smiling. Same as when you were a baby. No doubt when you roared and bellowed in your cot, your parents belted into the bedroom, tired, irritable, but anxious to soothe. But you can bet they cooed and cuddled and generally responded in the most satisfactory manner when you flashed them a gummy grin. Flirting works because it makes people feel good about themselves. And if you think of it this way you can flirt with anyone, even yourself.

A great flirter regards life as good fun. She loves to play, and tease. She isn't scared of people, of enjoying herself with them, whatever defences they put up. What man wouldn't want to get closer to a woman like that? She makes neurotic, self-doubting people relax and laugh at themselves. She talks to everyone – from the electrician to her boss — as if they're the most important people in the world, and wins their warmth and respect. She makes people feel good because life is more pleasant that way.

The opposite of a good flirter is a worrier. The worrier wouldn't dare flirt as it would present too much of an issue for her. Men scare her. Rejection scares her. Everything scares her. She's the kind of woman who looks at her feet, plays with her hair and is generally so uptight when conversing with a man that he feels a strong urge to book her into therapy and run out of the room. Meanwhile, the flirter enjoys herself. We all know a woman who flirts naturally, indiscriminately. She may not be gorgeous — but her vivacity makes her gorgeous. Resolve to see flirting as a way of life. Start with the postman. Then your boss. And your colleagues. And don't neglect the women in favour of the men. Have a nice day now...

How to Seduce Your Dream Man

Attention Grabbing for Daring Days

A) Spill your drink on him. Incidentally, comedian Vic Reeves met his wife this way so we know it's worked at least once. But go easy. You don't have to tip the entire glass of red wine over his Prada suit to get his attention. A splash on his shoes will do (but make sure they're not suede). If you reckon he's a tad particular about his appearance (see above) which in plain English means vain, a small splash will suffice. You want to get the balance right by spilling enough so that it's an issue, so he is forced into a conversation (of which more in a sec), but not too much that he is so utterly enraged at your abject stupidity he tells you to get lost. The ideal result of this delicate scenario is that a few splashes of red liquid splatter his jacket.

Aiming for his jacket is important because he can't just throw it in the wash (unless it is one of those very cheap polyester drip-dry ones, in which case he has no style and you may conclude he is not your type after all or he definitely needs you and you've found him not a moment too soon). Then you say 'I am sooo sorry'. Then pause while he huffs and swears then remembers his friends are watching and he isn't a sixth form girl and pretends he isn't too upset that you've stained his outfit. Then you sweetly say 'The least I can do is pay for you to have it dry-cleaned.' If at this point he refuses and means it, say 'Well, can I buy you a drink?' Otherwise, pause then add, 'Take my number' – *pause, dig around in pockets, grimace, find business card.* 'Give me a ring and I'll send you a cheque for the dry cleaning. I'm really sorry.' Then walk away. Don't hang around expectantly or it will be obvious it's a ruse. You want to be in control.

B) Bump into him accidentally on purpose so he spills his drink over himself – or over you. If he spills it over himself, see above for how to proceed. You have the additional option of offering to buy him another drink. If he spills it over you, he isn't going to feel remorse if he thinks it's your fault. So (and this requires coordination) you need to plan, rather like a pair of pickpockets. You squeeze past him and, at this exact moment, your girlfriend gives him a sharp jolt in the back then vamooses into the crowd before he spies her. Ideally, he will spill a small amount of booze on your black, sexy, but washable top and feel terrible about it...

C) Tap him on the shoulder and exclaim 'Mark!' (Or if you think this is too common a name, exclaim

How to Seduce Your Dream Man

'Orlando!') When he turns around you widen your eyes and gasp winningly, 'Sorry, from the back you look exactly like a friend of mine ... but from the front you look completely different!' The idea is to strike up a conversation. If he's worthwhile he'll muster up a playful response like 'better looking?' Some men swear that if a woman trots up to them and says 'Hi!' it's enough. But you've got to be lucky. 'Hi!' is all very well, but it isn't a great cue. Similarly, the 'Don't I know you' technique – it is clichéd and makes it easy for him to reply 'No' (if he's an oaf). The best strategy is to say something that makes it easy for him to catch the ball and run with it.

D) Drop loads of change on the floor. The key here is to go for it in a big way – squirrel away all your two pound coins first however – no need to take great risks here. But make a scene. Spill the contents of your purse from a great height. You want coins crashing, rolling, higgledy-piggledy all over the place, people staring, you want to manufacture the average Brit's worst nightmare. You want him to feel obliged to help you recover your pennies. This is a cinch for a man – he can be chivalrous at no cost to himself, he doesn't have to lift heavy bags, and he doesn't have to get his hands dirty changing tyres.

The Direct Approach for No-Nonsense Women

Wait until he trots off to the bar (i.e. away from his friends, as men live to make it difficult for their friends to score) then sidle up, on the pretext of buying a drink, and ask him any question you can think of. The object of this is not to be devastatingly witty – save that till later – it is to bring to his attention the fact that you exist. So, ask him anything – from the very plain, obvious but functional 'Do you have the time/a light?/both?' to the more daring but rather cute 'Is it hot in here or is it just you?' Some (American) experts advise sauntering up and saying 'I love your shirt, may I ask where you got it – I need to get a birthday present for my brother.' Fine if you can say it slinkily and without looking as if you know he knows you both know it's a great fat lie you've concocted in order to talk to him.

In the interests of research, a friend tested this line. The man in question looked at her in a raised eyebrow kind of way and she giggled. He then said 'That's just a line, isn't it?' She confessed and said 'Well, if you must know, my brother is ten!' – and he grinned and bought her a drink and – to date – they are very happy together. It's whatever you think will work with him.

The Even More Direct Approach

Perhaps you don't have the time or patience to play games. Still, wait till he is at a safe distance from his friends. Then – perhaps at the bar – say, 'I know you're with friends but I'd really like to buy you a drink. May I?' This approach – excessively polite, but not grovelling or apologetic – prompts a number of responses: the teasing 'Of course you may,' or (after appraising glance) 'Let me buy you a drink.' The drink line is less portentous than 'Would you like to go out with me?' (Hello? a second ago I didn't even know you existed) but effectively it means the same thing.

Hooray Note
I have it on good male authority that if a woman approached a man in this way, the only way he'd turn her down was if he was with his girlfriend – yawn, au revoir – or he was drinking with a friend he hadn't seen in ten years and whose death was imminent. And then – this is a direct quote – 'You'd regretfully say "Can you come back tomorrow, my friend's about to die – he'll be dead by five, can we have a drink at 6.30 – there's a pub I know near the hospital… "'

If however and more likely, he is drinking with friends he sees every week and who, despite their habits, seem destined for a reasonably long life – 'You'd ditch them in a shot and walk off with your thumb in the air because you've pulled.' Ah, so it's not exactly dignified for the woman then? Would he lose respect for her? 'No, you'd be thinking "Thank you for saving me the trouble of asking you. If only all women were like that."'

Bother Note
This Judas to the male sex adds, 'It does make you big-headed and think "She fancies me so I don't have to do so much."'

Our Verdict
You only have to stand behind some men in a queue and they think you're after them (well, you are, in a sense). So, what do you care? You've practically got a date! Also, even if he asked you first, the fact that you said 'Yes, I'd like a gin and tonic,' will also make him think, 'She fancies me … I've pulled.' At this stage, don't concern yourself about how far he thinks he's going to get with you, possibly tonight, just because you made the first move. The point is – the man you are intent on is sitting with you, gazing into your eyes and grinning like the Cheshire cat on Prozac. Admittedly, he is the one in control as he is more certain of your feelings than you of his. Let him enjoy his short-lived triumph. He is putty.

Childish but Effective Ways to Even Things Out

- Just as he's thinking 'I wish I'd changed the sheets in the last quarter,' you end the drink by kissing him demurely on the cheek, shoving your business card into his pocket, saying 'Thanks for the drink – give me a call,' and sashaying out of the door.
- Say 'Thanks for that – I really enjoyed it. But I'd better get back to my friends.' Then kiss him on the cheek – near the mouth, but on the cheek – and walk away. There is a 95% chance he will sheepishly wander over later – or if he's playing it safe, corner you when you are next at the bar – and ask for your number.

Personal Space Alert

However you wangled it, you and he are yakking. But don't stand too close to him. People get touchy about invasion of their personal space – it's partly why everyone is so growly on the tube. Invading someone's space is an aggressive, insensitive thing to do and it makes people hostile. Furthermore, men like to think of themselves as predators. So, if you are talking to him and you decide to stand three inches from his face before he has inched towards you, he may subconsciously think you are chasing him (absurd thought) and he may consciously feel a rise of irritation towards you. Let him be the one to step towards you. You don't need to move a muscle sweetie.

When You Know Who You Want: Stalking Lite

Engineer the meeting by research. Find out where he likes to hang out, and start hanging out there. Bribe a girlfriend, or a few to accompany you. Your goal should be to have fun irrespective of whether he turns up. Although he is the reason you are staking out the Pig & Pen, don't spend the entire night glancing over your shoulder. Get there relatively early so you can park yourselves at a conspicuous table, get the drinks in, and enjoy yourselves. This strategy gives you a double advantage: he will very possibly spot you first – indeed, nearly all men frequenting the pub will spy you from your superb attention-grabbing spot. When he does spy you, you will not resemble a myopic vulture, peering ravenously round the room (which always looks desperate and slightly sad). You will be laughing becomingly and (heheh) unselfconsciously with your gal pals over some impossibly witty remark...

Back down to earth – that said, men are almost unbelievably bad at spotting you when you want them to. Thus, each girlfriend, yourself included of course, will periodically leave the table to go to the toilet or order more drinks – in reality to scour the crowds in search of your prey, and report back.

Reeling Him In

Don't creep furtively into a room, it makes people want to smack you. Stride in like you own the place. Smile – not the village idiot grin, just a happy expression. Look into the room, rather than at the floor. Don't fiddle with your hair or clothes. If you need a prop, carry your bag or, if you must, your cigarette packet. If you walk in as though you are afraid of nothing and no-one, everyone – Mr Right included – will think 'She must be something special.' Whereas, if you slink in back to the wall like a criminal, you give him no incentive to come over. Body language like this shrieks 'Go away, leave me alone.'

And, however much it hurts, keep smiling. Most people don't smile because they're scared of being rebuffed. Big deal. You smile at a man, he doesn't smile back – oh no, the rest of your life is in tatters. So what. You had nothing to lose – he didn't smile back – he has an attitude problem – at least you find out now rather than a year on. The guy who's worth your time will smile back.

Whereas. If you walk into a room with a face as stern as a headmistress, he figures you look about as much fun as a headmistress – and not a kinky one, but an inner city comprehensive school headmistress whose study has just been set on fire for the third time this week. Men rarely assume a woman is shy. Instead they assume she's snooty and standoffish.

Smoking. Hmm. If he doesn't smoke himself he'll think it's gross. If he does, the entire habit becomes a seduction ritual (and this is a seduction book not a feature in the *Lancet* so although lung cancer, yellow teeth, and bad breath isn't sexy we'll refrain from stating the obvious). You ask him for a light, you clasp his hand to steady it as he flicks on his lighter, or does some fancy match-lighting manoeuvre which he perfected in his bedroom as a teen-ager when his parents were out, you blow the smoke out of the side of your mouth etc., etc. We're not condoning it, we're just acknowledging it exists.

Prompting an Exchange of Numbers

The best eventuality is not to offer him your number but to let him ask for it. Anyhow, by the end of your first meeting, he should know where you work, and your last name. If there has been no drink-spilling, make it easier for him to ask you for your number – lay the groundwork. You can do this by winding the conversation around to say, the book of the moment, then mentioning that actually there's a book you're far more keen to read, but haven't been able to get hold of. (Here, you name a book he probably owns, for example *Bravo Two Zero*. Just why you haven't been able to get hold of a very popular book is irrelevant, because if he wants an excuse to stay in touch, he'll grab it.)

You might wonder why you shouldn't leave it to him to just ask, but, and no disrespect to men, they are on the whole, supremely lazy. If anything is the remotest effort there is a chance they won't bother with it. Your goal is to smooth his path. If he isn't completely witless, he'll say 'I've got a copy. You can borrow that.' To which you reply (not too effusively, rather a judicious dollop of surprised gratitude), 'Oh, would you mind? That's so nice of you.'*

We're not yet home and dry. He might just be saying that for something to say. You'll realize this is the case if he then acts as if the subject is closed – i.e. no taking down of numbers to make it possible to phone and hand over the book. If this happens you dig out your trusty business card and say 'Call me at work when you find the book – I'll send a bike!' (This is a veiled reprimand – it makes him think that maybe you're not looking for an excuse to see him, indeed your life is so busy you'll send a courier.)

* I was going to suggest 'Would you mind ... that's really kind' – but it rhymes. Never a good idea, unless it's on purpose, and mostly not even then.

The Gentle Touch

Restrain yourself. It's not a great idea to – as the saying goes – be all over him. If you start stroking his cheek at the least provocation, clutching at his arm to emphasize your point, smacking him playfully on the chest when he says something funny, he will think 'She wants me – I'm in!' Plop! you have transferred all the power into his large head. Whereas, if you hold back, the power is all yours. The best strategy is to ration him to one touch on the pretext of emphasizing a point, possibly a light stroke on his hand (skin to skin – don't waste your electrifying touch on his jumper) and then not again.

That's it. This way, that single touch is memorable, significant, and – to borrow a Mills & Boonism – the sheer sexual promise of it will sear his skin and send the blood coursing through his veins (if it isn't already, in which case you've got problems). Touching him once keeps you in control, as he isn't sure whether you were merely emphasizing your point or trying to tease him (heheh) and is as confused as a chicken at a crossroad. He also wants more. The anticipation, the uncertainty, the I-want-what-I-can't-have mentality, the testosterone – all will fuse. He will be busting to touch you, and will be desperate, anxious for you to touch him again. When you say goodbye, kiss him on the cheek but near to his mouth. It will make him think...

Thinly disguised excuses to touch him plus a wisecrack or suggestive remark – should be used sparingly:

- You remove some fluff from his clothing (say something jokey like 'Oh, Gorillas In the Mist!' or he'll think 'I don't need another mother.')
- You remove a stray eyelash from his cheek (smile and whisper 'Make a wish.')
- You wipe a bit of food off his face (urk – but it's a very intimate, forward, and suggestive thing to do. Sensual perhaps).
- You touch him lightly on the back (someone's trying to squeeze past – say 'I didn't want you to get hurt.')
- You engineer a conversation about fitness and thus have an excuse to squeeze his bicep ('Flex for me darling, ooh, very hard... ')*

---

* Feel free to camp it up, mock, tease, lay it on thick – but distinguish what sort of man he is. Is he the shy man who thinks 'She couldn't possibly fancy me' or is he the macho, or conceited man who thinks the checkout lady fancies him because she asked him if he wanted cash back. Assess how highly aware he is of his own charms and proceed accordingly. If he's prone to Everyone Lusts After Me-Itis, ditch the flirtatious remarks – just touch him once or not at all and let him wonder. If he is the sort who only notices a hint if it hits him on the head with a large stick, you may have to put Julian Clary to shame.

When he Just Doesn't Get It

If he's ponderously slow at taking hints (this type does exist) you can hang around flicking your hair, licking your lips, flashing your bellybutton ring, and showing him your dolphin tattoo, and he won't get it. He'll think you're a fidgety woman who's being friendly. Admittedly, this type is as rare as a white tiger.

What Not To Do

Liane, 25, 'I met Marcus on the first day of college and thought he was beautiful. He had cut glass cheekbones, permanent five o' clock shadow, and very dark floppy hair. I did everything I could to make him realize I wanted to shag him senseless – and have a meaningful relationship too, of course. After dinner, I'd say "Anyone, come and have a coffee in my room? Marcus?" Or, "Anyone want to go to the bar? Marcus?" Or "A bunch of us are going to the cinema, open invitation. Marcus?" Sometimes he'd come, but other people would be there too and he'd never make a move. He did invite me to things too – sometimes people on his corridor would cook together on a Saturday night when the canteen was shut, and he'd ask me along.

But no singling out, no flirting. Eventually I gave up – he just wasn't on for it. Then, last year, we had a reunion, and as I was in another relationship and didn't mind what he thought, I said to him "You know I fancied you for the whole three years?" He was incredulous. He said, "If only I'd known, if only you'd let me know." I thought, "Short of sneaking into your room naked at 2am, sliding into bed with you and grabbing your penis, what more could I have done?"'

What to Do

With a hard case like this, the only way to make him realize you fancy him is to get tipsy at somewhere it's expected, like at a party, or get to the I-couldn't-care-less point where you come out with it. However, you lay your dignity on the line because there's nowhere to hide if he says, 'That's very sweet but I don't fancy you.' The more cowardly but safer ploy is to say teasingly, 'Did you know I had a crush on you once?' The realization churns slowly through his head and he thinks 'If she had a crush on me once, maybe she could again … ' This is a good ploy for the man you've known for a while – through work, college, or mutual friends – but with whom the right moment never arose.

If he has one brain cell, he'll say 'You did?' which is the cue for you to say carelessly, smilingly, 'Yeah, but you were never interested, so I gave up … ' His next remark – which requires at least two brain cells – should be 'Um, would you like to go out sometime?' After all, if you'd fed the line to him with a giant spoon, it couldn't be more apparent. If the baboon doesn't say what's expected, give him a fond kiss on the cheek and walk away. Let him stew. He most certainly will. You, meanwhile, get on with your life. You have nothing to be embarrassed about – men like this, unless they are weird, love to be told that someone fancies or fancied them. They review and revise their memories, and their self-esteem rockets. Chances are, he'll ask you out after thinking about it, unless he is:

■ in love with someone else, or
■ already aware of the fact but pretending ignorance because he isn't interested, in which case yah boo to him.

Let Them Come to You

In a Perfect World, you'd be sauntering around Sainsburys,
wondering if you should purchase the Pringles Cheezums
or the Family Pack of Dairy Milk or both, you'd reach
out to grab the Pringles first and zzzt! your arm brushes
against someone also reaching out for that selfsame tube of
Pringles and a tingle of electricity goes up your spine (and
other places). You look up, smiling, and see a vision – surely the prototype of manhood – and this gorgeous creature
is grinning back at you and (quick check) he has no wedding ring and (quick check again) his basket is full of single
man stuff: beer, ready-cook chicken korma, pork paté,
white bread, yes – and he says (in a voice that could melt
knickers) 'It's the last tube of Cheezums ... maybe we
could share them,' and breathily, huskily, you say, 'Maybe
we could ...' and he says, 'Then let me take you away
from all this,' and he picks you up ('Why, you're as light as
a, ah, Pringle!'), whisks you out of Sainsbury's (paying
first) and spirits you away in his tasteful car (a Nissan
Skyline in fact) to his oh so endearing bachelor flat
(scruffyish, but no black leather furniture or mounted
pictures of ex-girlfriends), and he has a beautiful grey cat

who purrs around your feet and he smiles and his eyes crinkle and he says 'She was abandoned, so I adopted her – she's called Titus Andronipuss' and then he pours some wine – Chateauneuf du Pape, actually – and you eat Pringles and you talk all night and you feel you've known him for ever – and it's like coming home, and he doesn't turn out to be a serial killer, and you kiss and it's the most erotic, amazing, headspinning experience you've ever had, and you can't believe it, and yes, he's got a job, he's successful, and he's intelligent, and he's got the right books on his shelves, and he has no dodgy opinions, he gets on great with his parents, and he's funny, and normal, but special and he's obviously mad about you and you have incredible sex and he's brilliant at it, and he's a lad and a feminist and his worst habit is picking his toes and you live happily ever after.

Infuriatingly – no offence to Sainsbury's – this doesn't happen very often. More likely you buy the Pringles and the Dairy Milk without incident (unless you count an old lady wheeling her trolley over your toe) and you return home alone, feast on both (the Pringles not the old lady), feel slightly sick, check your stomach side-on in the bathroom mirror to see if it's grown, and resolve to go to the gym tomorrow. So, although the loiter-in-supermarkets-and-find-a-man idea is cute, it has an average success rate of 0.001%. The same goes for libraries, bookshops, museums, and coffee shops. You can waste an awful lot of time and money and return home jittery with caffeine and laden with nice but non-essential books like *Cooking With Elvis* and *Speedy Tai Chi For Busy People* and no man. People in public places tend to be unfriendly or with friends. That means going to places where you're supposed to meet people – like a bar or disco. And the type of men you meet there are largely idiots. So, instead of the scattergun approach, you need to use the golden bullet. You host a singles party. Here are some tips:

- Plan the venue well in advance, preferably not in your home – at a funky venue, somewhere central.
- Issue invitations to all the single people you know – even those you don't normally mix with socially, say friendly business acquaintances. If they're female the rule is, they have to bring a single male friend, if they're male, they have to bring a single female friend – and lots of alcohol. If they want, those single people can invite their single friends. But absolutely no couples.
- Buy a bunch of plain white stickers and write a name on each. Each name is one of a pair, for example Bonnie/Clyde, The Queen/Prince Philip etc. Not everyone has to be a person – get as saucy as you like, for example Peephole/Bra, Crotchless/Knickers, then split into two piles.
- As every man enters, he is issued with a sticker from the male pile. As every woman enters, she is issued with a sticker from the female pile. The goal is to find your partner – the perfect excuse for everyone to mingle.

■ As you are on the door, you can issue yourself with a sticker, and when a delicious looking man comes in, slap the other half of your combo on his manly chest. If you want to be really sneaky, you can do several combinations for yourself – for example, if you are Apple, you can issue all the men you like the look of with names such as Crumble, Tart, Pie, Pie Bed, Of My Eye … my god, how many men do you want?

Smugnote
The joy is, you increase your circle of friends and your access to single men, and you get invited back to parties and you can host a singles party every couple of months should you wish – until Mr Right marches through the door.

Puffing up his Ego

The average man's ego is the size of Arizona, yet as delicate as a freshly baked soufflé. So proceed with caution. You think you're having a carefree chat about nothing in particular, you make a light-hearted remark and – ba-boom! his smile freezes on his lips and you feel a sudden chill – as if you just fell into a freezer cabinet. What did you do? Possibly you contradicted his idea of his identity. For example:

Juliette, 25: 'I met this guy through mutual friends, and we all started meeting up as a group. He was a sweet man, but with no flair – as I could see it. We were getting friendlier, until he said something that irritated me. It was something like "I'm a nutter!" I thought "Just because you wear wacky clothes that doesn't make you a nutter." So I said, "You seem perfectly sane to me." His face fell. As if that wasn't enough, the same night we were all going to a party and he came downstairs in what can only be described as a boiler suit. It was really odd – white with coloured squiggles on it. I think he thought it was wacky, but I burst out laughing and said "You look like Andy Pandy!" After that he ignored me. As if I cared!'

Fortunately, Juliette had no wish to date Andy Pandy – she's merely a handy example of how not to charm a man you fancy. You can figure out what he thinks of himself by what he says, does, and wears. If you reinforce his idea of who he is, he'll warm towards you. If you squash it, you dent his ego, and he resents you. We all harbour a little fantasy of who we are – and on a good day, indulge it. So, when you've glammed up, you're chatting to an admiring circle of males, they're laughing at your jokes, you see yourself – almost like an out of body experience – as a fun, sexy, popular woman. If another woman strolled up – ooh, let's say, Cameron Diaz, and the group's attention swung away from you to her, and you stood there like a plank while everyone fawned and she didn't attempt to include you in the conversation, unless you had an ego of steel, your perception of yourself as a fun, sexy, popular woman might falter a little. It shouldn't be like that, but it is.

Our perception of ourselves, apart from the weirdos with unshakeable self-esteem, wobbles according to how others behave towards us. Men may be less touchy, on the whole, than women but their self-perception can still be rocked. This certainly doesn't mean agreeing with every nonsense he comes out with, but when people are nervous they blurt out awful things – make sure that person isn't you. And watch your expression – wrinkling your nose and raising an eyebrow in response to his admission that he works for *Trout & Salmon* magazine is as crushing as saying 'Well, someone has to.'

He thinks he's on his way to becoming editor of *The Times*. He also knows how hard it is to get into journalism these days. He's also pretty chuffed because he loves fishing. He secretly thinks it's glamorous work and he likes to use all the terminology such as 'urgent deadline,' 'filing copy' etc. – and looks on himself as a dashing young Hunter S. Thompson. You have made him feel like a no-hoper berk who can't get a proper job. And you thought you were gently teasing him or – (a million times worse) being honest. Oops.

Dealing with his Friends

Part I

This includes not making him look foolish in front of them. The worst thing you can do is to correct him,* either on his grammar ('Surely fewer people not less people'), a geographical certainty ('I'm afraid you're confusing Bucharest with Budapest'), or a film fact ('I think you'll find that Steve McQueen was Coppola's first choice to play Willard in *Apocalypse Now* – he was succeeded by Al Pacino, then shooting began with Harvey Keitel, only for Coppola to ditch him in favour of Martin Sheen two weeks later.') Actually, blowing him out of the water with your expert knowledge of what's traditionally thought of as a guy's film is pretty damn cool. You'll either impress him into bed or make him want to throttle you.

However, on the whole, no one fancies a pedant, unless they look like Liz Hurley or Ralph Fiennes, and even then it detracts from their charm. Furthermore, no one likes to be made to look like a prat in front of an audience. Men

---

* Unless you are having a sexual tension contest – see 'Sparring' below.

are particularly touchy. They hate to lose face in the presence of their friends because they are driven by the concept of competing. (Same goes for women but we're more subtle about it.) Their status within their peer group is essential, and while there are two things he can pretty much control to show this – his job and his car – the woman is the rogue element. You highlight this by showing him up in front of his pack and – while they crease up with laughter – he hates you.

Part II

It's also important to stand up to his friends because if they dislike you they'll let him know it, and men are susceptible to what their friends think. First, this means refusing to let them upset you even if they are a bunch of Neanderthals whose idea of culture is setting their farts alight. So, when you and your intended are at a crucial bonding moment and one of his pals – named Rozza or Dazza – sticks his great grinning beerfumey face between you and sings 'Alright mate, trying to getcha leg over?' your understandable instinct is to pull out a gun and shoot him dead. Instead, you sit there puce and prim with embarrassment while your intended tells Dazza where to stick it. Thanks to Dazza, the beautiful moment lies in tatters, its brains splattered over the pub floor.

Your goal is to soothe your man's mortification while showing Dazza that his remarks cut no ice with you. Raise an eyebrow, and say, 'If he is it's fine with me.' Then wink at Mr Right and change the subject. Never mind if this is not the case. You can slap his hands away later. Whatever, he will appreciate your unruffled handling of the situation. Resist the temptation to slag off Dazza at length. Even though your intended has spent his entire youth and early adulthood trying to get one up on Dazza, he likes him. Dazza is a plonker but he is also a mate. You, however, are the new kid on the block, so don't push it. Although, if all his friends are like Dazza that may be a worrying clue to his own personality.

What Not To Say on a First Meeting

- 'I'll stick to orange juice, I've got terrible period pain, really heavy flow, it feels like it's dragging my whole uterus out of my body, I get really bloated, it's agony, alcohol makes it worse.'
- 'Yeah, that's my plan – marry someone rich then retire ha ha!'
- 'My ex, what a psycho, he once locked me in a cupboard for three hours because he said I was freaking him out by nagging him too much, god I hate men like that, what a loony, sometimes, if he ran out of clean underwear he'd wear the same pair of pants two days in a row, he'd turn them inside out, disgusting, I mean, can you believe that? And sometimes when he breathed his nose squeaked.'
- 'Well, Bunnee-Pinkums sleeps on the pillow, and Wuffer-Puffer sleeps next to her – then BaaLamb gets at least a foot of the bed to herself, also she doesn't get on very well with Mr Whisker so they have to be separated… '.

- 'Well, as my mother says.'
- 'Oh 30 at least! I was a late starter but once I got going, well, ha ha, there was no stopping me, let's see, Mark, blond well-built if you get my drift, but it didn't last — the relationship I mean, he personally could go on and on, then there was Luke, tall, slightly overweight but something to hold on to, know what I mean!'
- 'You don't look very strong.'
- 'So you went out with her for how long? And what's her name? And what does she look like? And what does she do? And was she good in bed? And how often do you see her? And where does she live? And is she going out with anyone? And do you still fancy her? And is she prettier than me?'
- 'I didn't get on with my father, you see, so after the anorexia, I was in and out of clinics, I suppose I was improving but when my aunt died I just lost it, I started cutting myself — nothing serious, just a few scratches but it's a downhill slope, so I was seeing a psychiatrist, but I didn't think much of him so I was referred to someone else, he was much better, but then … '
- 'Accountancy? – poor you!'
- 'How much do you earn?'
- 'Oh I dunno. I just feel (sigh) as if I'm a bit of a failure. I mean (sigh) I hate my job, and I'd really like to do something more interesting and like, maybe, travel a bit, but (sigh) that means I'd need to find lodgers and (sigh) I don't know if I'd get my old job back when I came back

How to Seduce Your Dream Man

– I mean, I know I said I hate it, and I do, but (sigh)
well, it's so hard, y'know.'
■ 'Ideally, I'd like to be engaged by the end of this year.'

Quick One
Laugh at his jokes and know a few of your own.

Sparring

Otherwise known as sexual tension, very common in popular romance where story is as follows: girl meets boy, boy and girl irritate the hell out of each other, boy and girl kiss thanks to surplus of energy caused by adrenaline, boy and girl go back to irritating each other, boy and girl realize they actually are magnetically attracted to each other and the reason for all their squabbles is because they are fighting their feelings ... ooh, it makes the passion so much more *passionate*.

So tease him, bait him, disagree with him but do it light-heartedly — best topics for flirtatious disagreement are TV, celebrities, music, and anything else fluffy and fun. If he's not a twerp with no sense of humour he will rise to the challenge (ahem). The suggestions in Puffing Up His Ego still stand because there's a difference between teasing him and emasculating him.

Keep away from politics, feminism, religion and other potentially disastrous topics because you may end up red faced and screeching at him, which isn't seductive even if he does deserve it. Men have an infuriating tendency of writing off women who are beating them in an argument as 'Over-emotional.' If he implies as much, he's either a deadbeat or trying to wind you up. No doubt you'll be able to judge...

Perfecting the 'Come Hither' Look

Ideally, you shoot him a look that makes his insides jellify. Such a look takes perfecting, so practise on a trusted and good-humoured male friend. After all at some point you have to make eye contact, so you'll want it to be memorable. For all you know, every time you do make eye contact with a potential man you pull a wide-eyed expression like someone who has just sat on a pin, or blink furiously like a short-sighted snowy owl. Check with your friend who – if he is a friend at all – will suggest modifications. Cultivating the alluring look may take longer than you think because much of the time you and your pal will be doubled up on the floor weeping with laughter. The look that sends an arrow straight into his heart and groin should be coy, brazen yet innocent, from under the eyelashes. Don't flutter them though. Let him acknowledge you. Then hold his gaze for a second longer than is demure, then look away. Five seconds later, look back and smile.

Sealing Deal Note

If he has any initiative, he may hold up his drink as a 'Can I get you one?' sign and wend his way over. If not, engineer it so that you bump into him at some point. If he looks as though he'd like to start a conversation but is tongue-tied say something simple like 'You have a nice smile.' It isn't Shakespeare but it's good enough. But we digress. We're talking alluring looks, and — once you have secured his attention — the way to keep it is to focus on him. Don't stare fixedly at his face like a cat watching a budgerigar, but do pay attention. Don't look over his shoulder. It pisses people off. It's insulting. It makes him feel as if he's a stopgap until something better comes along. Men are attracted to women who make them feel special.

Make Him Want to Touch You

Texture – it's *soo* important. So ensure that:

- Your hair is soft and shiny. Ditch sticky, lacquery sprays – think ahead – if at some point he runs his fingers through your hair you don't want them to jam.
- You wear at least one tempting material – velvet, cashmere, thin cotton – don't overdo it and go out looking like a fluffy bunny.
- If you have good skin, wear as little foundation as possible – he'll want to stroke your cheek.

Quick One

Figure out what he likes about you and play on it, but not too much – you don't want to become a frightening yoof TV-presenterish caricature of yourself. However some men, in their innocence, give away what they like about the look of you in the first five minutes. And you'll want to capitalize on that. So:

- What he says: 'You look Italian, or Spanish.'
- What he means: You look exotic, exciting, interesting.

- What you say: 'Well, I speak Italian'*'My family are originally from Sicily.'**
- What you don't say: 'Nah sorry, Wolverhampton born and bred.'

- What he says: 'You have a filthy laugh.'
- What he means: I bet you're a right tiger when you get going.

- What you say: 'That's not the half of it darling (laugh).'
- What you don't say: 'Oh no, it just sounds like that today because of my laryngitis.'

- What he says: 'You have very expressive hands.'
- What he means: You seem an enthusiastic, lively, sensual person.

- What you say: 'That's what my ex-boyfriend used to say.'

* Don't say this if the only words you know in Italian are *penne arrabiata*. If you do speak Italian it's worth about 50 points – in manspeak: 'A bird who speaks Italian, fwaor!'

** Again, would be nice if it were true, but if it's not, and he asks too many questions, explain that your great-great grandfather whose surname was ah, Barberi, emigrated to Wolverhampton and the name Barberi then got anglicized to er Horncastle. Worth about 30 points – in manspeak: 'A bird with mafia connections ...'

- What you don't say: 'That's what my flute tutor says.'

- What he says: 'You look the sporty type.'
- What he means: You have a great body – I bet you can go on and on.

- What you say: 'Well, I surf and kickbox. It's more for fun than exercise.'
- What you don't say: 'It's all down to hard work – I don't eat junk food, and I'm teetotal, and I won't drink caffeine, honestly it's so bad for you, it's been linked with cancer, and I do the Mr Motivator workout every morning and twice a day at weekends.'

How to Seduce Your Dream Man

Don't Play Dumb

Truth is, playing dumb does attract men. It attracts gooberish idiots who are so stupid and insecure they feel threatened by a woman with a brain and a few opinions. If you twirl your hair around your finger, bat your eyelashes, giggle inanely at anything he says, and come out with stuff like 'Robin Cook – oh, is he the one who presents *Ready, Steady, Cook*? – oh right! Oh, I'm getting confused, I hate politics it's so complicated ... I prefer to leave it to the men, seems funny to have women politicians, all that shouting ... oh yes I would like another drink ... ooh I get all tipsy on a glass of white wine ... maybe something else but I don't know what, you choose!' This sort of man will be sniffing around you like a terrier around a lamp post. And he'll have the same degree of respect for you.

A thick man is attracted to women who play dumb because he assumes they're easy to take advantage of – 'Ooh, what are you doing, you naughty boy?! ooh go on then!' – and are no threat to Thicko's own limited intelligence. If you do have a sizeable brain and are in fact a high-powered career woman, business executive, or whatever, yet like to play the silly ikkle girl because it is an easy way to seduce a man, you are playing a foolish game. Thicko will be most displeased to find you are in fact a smart woman who knows the names and job titles of every person in the Cabinet and the Shadow Cabinet, doesn't take any crap, has a highly paid job and is well-respected, and hates ironing. He's not interested in what you say, want, or think. All he wants is some arm candy who's a good shag.

Whereas, a man worth nabbing is proud of your achievements, loves to hear what you have to say, is interested in your opinions, and likes women. He finds any excuse to boast about you to his friends – not 'My chick is 34DD' but 'New York? My girlfriend's just been to New York on business, just got promoted, yeah, company car – BMW Z3 – the lot, she's in charge of a massive department, was headhunted the other day.' Your brilliance reflects on him, it doesn't detract from him.

A man worth nabbing doesn't say things like 'Chuh! Women bloody drivers!' or 'Huh! Typical woman, always nagging!' or 'Women! why do they bother with an education – they only come out and start having babies!' Any man who says something like this is terrified of independent assertive women because secretly, although he'd never admit it even to himself, he knows they're brighter, sassier, and smarter than he is, and, essentially, wouldn't touch him with a barge pole and surgical gloves. The point? If you want to bring Mr Right to heel, tell it like it is. Voice your valid, informed opinions like a grown up, and buy him a drink.

How to Seduce Your Dream Man

Cultivate Your Sense of Fun

This is different from having a small stock of high quality –
and one or two really awful – jokes. A sense of fun doesn't
mean barking out a series of terrible puns or cracking one-
liners, it means relaxing a little. Some women are condi-
tioned to be good girls, which means they find it hard
to chill out. A little headmistressy voice inside them tells
them going to a football match is a bad idea because it
means they can't wear their suede boots, their hair might
get wet because it looks as though it's going to rain, and
there's no filter coffee available. Men don't like uptight
women who are scared to have fun, who won't have an ice
cream eating competition because they're watching their
weight. 'Watching my weight' is surely the most tedious
concept in the world and to a man it spells boredom.

A woman with a sense of fun does:

- accept a knickerbocker glory eating fest (first one to eat
  three is the winner)
- race him to the top of the hill
- and roll down it*

* Do all you can to surreptitiously check it's dogpooh-free.

- have snowball fights
- occasionally stay out till five am on a week night
- drink him under the table
- know the offside rule or, at least, Jamie Redknapp's position
- love going to the fair
- build sandcastles.

A woman with a sense of fun does not:

- insist on staying in a five star hotel on every weekend away
- sulk all evening and the next day if beer gets spilt on her trousers
- say things like 'Your friends are so immature'
- stay till the bitter end of a terrible film because 'We paid for it, we may as well'
- hate to get her hands dirty
- turn down a night out at a groovy restaurant because 'I'll break my diet'
- tell him not to mess up her hair
- cry if she misses her train
- freak out when she looks under his bed and finds a copy of *Playboy*.

Learn to Mix Like a Pro

Maximize your chances by plonking yourself in all the right situations. Parties. Premieres. Trendy new bars. Dinner parties. Of course, there are limits – one American magazine once suggested hanging around disaster areas because they were bound to be teeming with hoards of hunky handsome heroic firemen! The catch – which was overlooked – is how to come on to a guy who is rescuing an injured baby from a bombed out building? What exactly is the protocol here? To tap him on the shoulder and say: 'This might be a bad moment but I just wanted to say, red looks really great on you.' Or, when questioned by a police officer on the reason for your loitering presence 'I was hoping that, after you've finished shunting out all the bodies, you could direct me to the nearest cafe – preferably a trendy one with squishy sofas and free newspapers – and maybe even join me.'

Point is, when you find Mr Right you don't want him to think you're a psychopath. Unless you're a paramedic, your presence is an inconvenience, an embarrassment and possibly an offence. So let's forget disaster areas for now, and concentrate on the real world. Say you're invited to a party, and it is going to be teeming with delicious men. You do not want to come home mopey and deflated because although you saw someone you liked you didn't dare approach him, and some other unremarkable woman poached him proving that he was free and he may very well have been willing. You have to swallow your fear of interraction with groups of strangers, swan in there, and work the room. A few tips:

- Turn up with a friend – it stops you looking and feeling like a spare part.
- Avail yourselves of a drink (you have a good chance of striking up a conversation over the nibbles).
- Greet the host/hostess (superb because she/he can introduce you to people).
- Find a good vantage point with your friend and survey the room.
- If you see someone you know – male or female – approach them. If they're in a group which looks impenetrable, stand beside them and continue chatting to your friend. At some point, make eye contact with the person you know, smile, and if they smile back you have your chance – lean over, kiss them hello, and introduce your friend. If this person has any social grace at all, he/she will either introduce you to the rest of their group, or excuse themselves from their group and talk to you.
- If he/she introduces you to the group, say 'Hello' and shake everyone's hand. This may seem a little formal

(you judge if it is completely inappropriate) but a good firm handshake registers with people. If someone shakes your hand, looks you in the eye and says 'Hello, I'm so-and-so' you may forget their name immediately but you cannot ignore them. Whereas if they stand there awkwardly and give you a bashful nod and mumble something, why should you make any attempt to include them?

- If the person you know leaves the group to talk to you – great. No doubt they know people you don't, which doubles your chance of meeting someone new.

- If either your friend or you manages to engage a likely candidate in conversation, make a pact not to get huffy.

- If you really cannot see one single person you know, scour the room to see which group looks the least threatening. Then bluff your way into it. This does require nerves of steel – but if you can stand it, march up, make eye contact with the kindest-looking person, and say in a strong voice, 'Mind if we join you? I'm Blah, this is Blah, we don't know a soul here, and out of everyone you look like you're having the most fun!' Say it with conviction even if your sphincter is contracting as you speak – if you sound upbeat, and reasonably sane, people will be more welcoming. Even if one or two members of the group are sniffy, there is usually one sympathetic person who feels obliged to be friendly. Pretend you're acting a part in a film, say a Meg Ryan role – chirpy, unabashed, immune to cool glances.

- Once you've infiltrated the group, listen to the drift of their conversation and don't butt in and/or try to dominate it. Then, after a few minutes, speak up, preferably to express your agreement with the person who has just spoken and adding a salient point. Good luck.
- If you can't barge in cold, grab a tray of cheesy wotsits and offer them round. Er, only if it's a private party. Not if it's a book launch with professional caterers.

If none of the above appeals and you still can't figure out how to approach the one you think you love, check his finger for a ring and his close proximity for a girlfriend, then pinch his bottom. When he whirls around, you stage an Oscar-worthy performance: 'Oh. No. I am sooo sorry – I thought you were someone I knew. I am so embarrassed!' Please God he has a sense of humour and doesn't slap a lawsuit on you (don't try this one in the US).

Hog Him

Once you have secured his attention, minimize every other predator's chances. This means, if possible, manoeuvring it so that you face the room and he faces the wall. Thus, he is less likely to be distracted for the simple reason that few people enter his line of vision, and the majority of guests can only see his back. Anyhow, he shouldn't need to keep an eye on anyone else as he's talking to you.

Don't Vie for his Attention

Sometimes events don't go to plan. You are merrily chatting away to him, he seems entranced and is laughing in all the right places when another woman bowls up 'Tony/Mark/Matthew daaarrr-ling! How aarrre you? Mwa! Mwa!' She tactically ignores you, gives a stiff nod when he introduces you, and proceeds to monopolize him, practically clawing at his chest. You have a choice. You could of course start a vicious verbal battle – you and she fighting for his attention, interrupting each other, shooting each other snide looks, gabbling, babbling, pawing, feeling stupid and childish – while he looks on in slightly smug amusement and thinks he's it. (In the circumstances even Mr Right can be forgiven for this assumption.) Well, you're not going to pander to his ego or to Mwa Mwa's need to slight every woman she regards as a threat. It reduces you to beggar status – 'Oh *pleeeeze* choose meeee' – it is undignified and you're better than that.

The smart woman cuts in within, say, two minutes of Mwa Mwa's arrival, says loudly, 'Tony, lovely to meet you but there are a million people I should say hello to – say goodbye to me before you go,' and leans forward to kiss him while accidentally on purpose treading heavily on Mwa Mwa's toe. Then she swans off. Walking away doesn't mean you're giving up. It shows him that you rate yourself, and you're not just there for the taking.

It also shows your contempt for Mwa Mwa and highlights the fact that she is a pretty shallow waste of space. Mwa Mwa has novelty value – she's cute enough to flit around, talk entertaining nonsense, and flirt wildly – but dig deeper and she has nothing terribly interesting to say and, in truth, Mr Right finds her a bit much. Five minutes after you've gone he'll be missing you. If he was interested, your 'If you want me come and get me' behaviour will have stoked that interest – men still love a challenge. Ten minutes later, he will probably unpick Mwa Mwa's claws from his arm and come looking for you...

Truth Notes

A) It has to be said that on rare occasions, after you've walked off, he and Mwa Mwa kiss passionately and go home together. In which case – the man has truly terrible taste, but, and but is all that can be salvaged from the situation – at least you preserved your dignity. If he really wanted you, he would have shaken off Mwa Mwa and come and found you. By sticking to him like an agoraphobic leech you would not have won him. He knew who he preferred at the start of the evening and no amount of vying would have changed his mind. You would merely have made yourself feel foolish as it became obvious that he preferred Mwa Mwa to you. You lost nothing. Na-teeng!

B) Ideally, when Mwa Mwa tries to butt in, Mr Right will make it clear enough by his body language (touching you on the arm, looking at you when he speaks, asking you what you think etc.,) that he will not stand any rudeness from her because he likes and, very likely, prefers you.

C) However, even the sweetest man can be so awed by the attentions of two females (a common male fantasy as if you didn't know) that he just wants to sit back and let them claw it out. Which is why note b) is a relatively rare occurrence.

Never Assume

Assuming can put a man right off you. It is a tad offensive
— just as you'd be offended if the cheeky sod thought just
because you were chatting to him you wanted to get into
his Y-fronts. So, know this: just because a man is friendly,
doesn't mean he's on for it. Let's face it, he probably
is, judging from experience but we'll try not to make
generalizations. It's arrogant and it can be off-putting, so
whatever the situation don't be over-flirtatious from the
off. Rather — build up at your leisure.

Real Life, Real Assumption

Tabitha, 24 'I was in a bookshop and I was trying to find a book and I didn't have its exact title. One of the male assistants was really helpful. He was very friendly, cute, and very patient. I said quite innocently, "I've struck lucky with you!" meaning I felt lucky to have found someone so helpful in assisting me to find the book I wanted. He retorted "No you haven't!" As if! The cheek!'

Mirroring

Sly way of putting him at ease – you reflect his movements. It will help him arrive at the fortuitous conclusion that you two are in harmony, and possibly, meant to be. So if his arms are dangling at his side, relax yours, don't cross them. (Crossing your arms is a bad habit anyway because it is closed off and defensive – it signals that you are ill at ease and/or would prefer to be left alone, even if you don't realize it.) If you and he are sitting at a table and he leans forward, you should lean forward too. If you lean back, it suggests you wish to maintain your distance.

No need to be mechanical about it – or you turn into his brattish little sister who used to mimic everything he did or said 'Mum! what's for tea?' ... 'Mum! what's for tea?!' 'Oh shut up Angela!' 'Oh shut up Angela!' 'Just leave me alone!' 'Just leave me a- owww!' So, moderation is the key. If he laughs at something he's said, help him out with a chuckle. But every time he takes a sip of his drink, you don't have to follow suit – too slavish and he'll think you're a fruitcake.

Ways to Distinguish the Wheat from the Chaff

Or – sussing out who's an idiot and who's a nice guy disguised as an idiot.

Opening Remarks

- Boo: he's said, 'What do you do?' You tell him and he says, 'Really, well that's funny because I ... and I ... when I etc., etc.'

- Hooray: he's said, 'What do you do?' You tell him and he says, 'Really, that sounds interesting, how did you?' etc., etc.

- Why?: if he's really interested in you he won't immediately turn everything you say into an excuse to bark on about himself.

Appearance

- Boo: he's wearing a home-knitted jumper which – amid the garish pattern – is smattered in egg-stains.

- Hooray: he's wearing a scruffy un-ironed shirt and his trousers have seen better days.
- Why?: anyone over the age of 14 is too old to wear jumpers knitted by granny in a public place. Strongly suggests he is immature and – judging by the egg stains – can't be bothered to look after himself and needs mothering. Scruffiness however, is excusable – that's just bloke nature. As long as his clothes are clean.

Smell

Boo: slight whiff of BO.

Hooray: little heavy on the aftershave.

Why?: with modern plumbing and a vast range of sanitary products on the market he has no excuse to smell bad. Shows a shocking lack of self-awareness and selfish disregard for other people. Too much aftershave: doesn't necessarily mean he's a smooth cad, who of course would be wearing just the right amount. Possibly a little insecure and out on the pull. That's all you need to know, surely?

Hair

- Boo: flamboyant sideburns and slightly bouffed.
- Hooray: shockingly short.
- Why?: any man with showoffy sideburns is dealing with some issue you don't want to be any part of – either he is bitter at taking his parents' advice and becoming a lawyer rather than a rock star or he is insecure with his

masculinity and obsessed with the concept of balding and thinks no one will notice his bare pate if he covers his face with bumfluff. Bouffing is equally bad news (Michael Flatley – need we say more?) Short however is, on the whole, good, even if it isn't flattering. Either he has a refreshing lack of vanity (doesn't know a salon tragedy when he sees one) or has confronted his receding hairline in a healthy, stylish way. Consider the alternative: a comb-over.

Quick One
Try and show some interest in his car.

Posture

Great posture is a rare thing, because when you see someone who has it, you sit up and take notice. That's the plan anyway. You walk into a room with your supersonic posture and at least half the men present are going to think 'Wow – who's she?' Women who slouch, making themselves look like the Hunchback of Notre Dame's young cousin, do themselves a grand disservice. If you slouch you look defeated, submissive – as if the world is too much for you. Whereas if you stand upright you look serene, in control, not to mention slimmer and more elegant. It also enhances the shape of your bosom. You look as if you're worth knowing.

Incidentally standing upright is not the same as arching your back and sticking your chest out like a page three stunna. Also – when, say, you're standing at the bar – try not to sink all your weight on to one leg. If you stand firmly on both you look far more confident. You're also less likely to hunch.

How to Check your Posture

Stand up and relax your arms by your sides. Then bend your forearms 90 degrees as if you were going to clap.

Then, twist your palms round until they're facing outwards (feels fairly uncomfortable) and bring your arms down to your sides again. That is the position your shoulders should be in – your natural posture – how you were designed. If they don't stay in that position when you relax, your posture could do with improvement.

How to Improve your Posture
Sorry, but it means getting off the sofa. Pilates and/or the Alexander Technique is the answer. Pilates is a series of slow movements which exercise muscles deeply but do not stress them. It focuses on strengthening your stomach and back – and it is essential for your torso to be strong to support you and give you good alignment. The Alexander Technique teaches you how to improve your balance, co-ordination and movement, release tension and regain your natural poise. Men, unless they are athletes, do not tend to be terribly graceful – and they appreciate women who are. We're not talking about Jane Austenish grace and ability to play the pianoforte and sing sweetly at the same time, we're talking a slinky liquidity of movement. So relax – you don't have to drink tea with your little finger extended.

Quick One
Beat Him at Pool

Knickerless Tip

Forget to wear your knickers. He should start wondering and thinking evil thoughts. He'll enjoy driving himself crazy trying to work out if, maybe you're wearing a thong or nothing at all. If you wear a clingyish skirt or dress (not too short, we're being alluring not issuing an open invitation), if he has eyes in his head they will be drawn to your figure and he will notice, because he's a man, an absence of knickerline.

Real Life, No Knickers

Natascha, 25: 'I was dancing with a guy at a club, and he put his hands on my hips and suddenly he said "You're not wearing any knickers are you?" It was obvious – I'll let you guess how – that he was really turned on by this.'

Be an Ace at Small Talk

Know how to mastermind it. Get the balance between asking questions, being a good listener, and talking yourself. A few suggestions:

■ Don't finish his sentences for him.
■ Don't nod like a nodding dog as if you're desperate for him to hurry up and stop talking.
■ Although men like to talk about themselves there is a difference between asking questions and interrogation so,
■ don't be too nosy – even if you disguise it with nice words it's still nosiness, for example, 'I hope you don't mind me asking, but how much would you pay for a flat like that?'
■ If you want to draw him out, ask open-ended questions – for instance, if he says he's just been to the US on holiday, a smart woman would say 'How exciting, which bit? Did you have a nice time?' Then follow up with 'What did you do?' Thus giving her talking partner permission to expand. A bad conversationalist would shut him up before he's even started by saying, 'I go to the US quite often on business' – which effectively puts a great big

verbal bar in the way of him opening up about him because you force him (if he has any social nouse whatsoever) to ask about you: 'Oh right. What do you do?'

- Also, if possible, try to avoid closed questions that elicit a one-word answer. Ask open questions that provoke an emotional response. For example rather than say 'Do you like *The Sweeney?*' ('Yes') Ask 'Why do you like *The Sweeney?*' (Where shall I begin?)

- Don't put wit above the conversational flow. For example he says 'I'm feeling very smug – I'm the best man at a wedding this weekend – nothing to wear, walked into Oswald Boeteng, amazing suit, reduced to half price, flash of the card and I'm all set!' You could say 'Sounds gorgeous – whose wedding?'* Or you could say 'Ah, but does it fit you?!'**

- Talk about yourself but if he asks you a question you don't want to answer, don't. Just laugh and say nothing. Or, say 'None of your business sweetie.'

- Don't ramble on to fill a silence. Some men keep quiet on purpose to gain the upper hand. Don't fall for such a low-down trick. You're likely to say something silly and it makes you look nervous. If you've said what you want to say, shut up.

---

* Reasonable, polite question which gives him the opportunity to say 'My brother/close friend etc' and for you to ask further leading questions like 'How do you feel about that?'

** Stupid, smug-faced clever-dick rhetorical question that isn't particularly funny and brings the conversation to an undignified halt.

Be Tough Against Rejection

What's the worst thing that can happen? You think he's up for it – you've been flirting shamelessly all night, he's been giving you all the signs – yet when you say 'So, uh, do you want to meet up sometime?' He steps back, looks at you aghast, claps his hands loudly and shouts 'Everyone! Guess what! This woman here (points finger, everyone stares) thinks I want to go out with her and I don't!' Then, everyone in the room laughs uproariously at you because you fancied him and he didn't fancy you back so obviously you had ideas above your station, and what makes you think you're so special etc., etc.

When someone rejects us, this is how it can feel. Instead of thinking 'More fool you,' we wonder what's wrong with us. But, 'More fool you' should be the stock response inside your head. We won't pretend that rejection is anything other than one of the most misery making things in the world. But if you want to nab Mr Right, dealing with rebuffs from Mr Wrong in a positive way is essential.

First, establish why he may have rejected you:

- He doesn't know you but he thinks you're not right for him.
- He's going out with someone else.
- He does know you, but he thinks you're not right for him.
- He doesn't fancy you.

Peptalk

- He doesn't know you – so he's not rejecting you as a person; he doesn't know the wonder of you.
- It's not personal – he's already spoken for. Pity the woman he's going out with that he has to flirt excessively with others to satisfy his ego.
- If he does know you: he thinks the two of you would not be suited as a couple. It doesn't mean he thinks you're worthless/boring etc., it means he doesn't think you're right for him. He's entitled to his opinion, and maybe he's right. None of us are right for lots of people – even, regretfully, Matt Dillon or Matt Le Blanc. Even if you envy the great relationship your good friend has with her fiancé, you wouldn't want to marry him.
- While many men in this world fancy Kate Moss, some men think 'Ugh – too skinny, pointy nose,' which is to say, whatever you look like, not every man in the world is going to fancy you. It's nothing personal, it's just reality. Think of the men who did/do fancy you.

Extra Note

Why should this man's decision have any bearing on your self-estimation? If you feel American-minded enough, write a list of, say, five wonderful things people have said to you that made you feel great. What he thinks doesn't change you in any way. You are exactly the same person you were this morning – you are not, suddenly, a worse person.

If he rejects you in a demeaning way, he's confirmed he's a moron. Excellent – once you have smoothed your ruffled feathers, this will hasten your recovery as you will be forced to admit to yourself that he's a berk. Because, unless you have been stalking him (stalking lite doesn't count) or behaving badly yourself – there is no excuse for nastiness. It doesn't reflect on you, it reflects on him. We are only spiteful to people if something they are/have/do makes us uncomfortably aware of something we lack.

Plain Example

When Susanna, 25, announced her engagement, her colleagues were thrilled for her. Except one person, Martine. Martine's response was 'You're mad. You're making a mistake. You're far too young to get married.' My, my, a confident person might have thought – why so touchy? Susanna, however, didn't think 'What's wrong with her that she isn't, like a normal friend, pleased for me?' She thought, 'Maybe I am too young.' She confided in her good friend Laura who asked for a little information about Martine. Susanna: 'Well, she's separated from her husband, who left her for another woman.' Hmm. Why is there no mystery here?

The Point
If a man rejects you in an unnecessarily cruel way (for example he reacts snidely if you ask him to dance, your most dignified reply is a cool 'There's no need to be rude.') – his behaviour suggests *he* has a problem, as do the following scenarios:

- He just doesn't call = weak, cowardly, juvenile.
- You ask him to dance, he says 'not with you' = insecure about masculinity, immature, has to make himself look 'hard' and 'big' by making other people look small, miniscule penis (medical terminology: matchstick dick).
- You make conversation, he replies in monosyllables = socially inept, possibly badly brought up, shallow, vain.
- He leads you on, after weeks you realize he's not interested = control freak, emotional hang-ups, cold nature.
- You sleep with him once, he slags you off = his pathetic bedroom performance has never been challenged, you as a woman who knows what she wants and doesn't put up with less makes him aware of his inadequacies, he has a mental age of ten, strong women scare him because he's weak and insecure.

Overall Verdict
Thank him for saving you from wasting your time.

Peptalk
Every time some dufus says no, you're one man nearer to the perfect one who says 'I like everything about you, please may I keep you?'

There are a squillion toads out there and probably only one-tenth of a squillion princes. The joyous thing is, you only need *one* prince. Even better, some toads, when they meet the right woman, turn into princes.

There's no such thing as 'All the good men are spoken for' – some wonderful men, like some wonderful women, meet their perfect partner aged 32 or 38, not 22.

Get Friends on the Lookout

They will fix you up with a gargoyle or two, but number three might just be the one. Also, they have a vague idea of the kind of man you like. Oh, and be gracious about the gargoyles or your friends might go into a huff and stop bothering.

Quick One
Wear exquisite underwear as often as possible (this is, of course, for the days you're not eschewing knickers). It boosts your confidence. Whether anyone sees it is irrelevant – it makes you feel innately sexier. It's no coincidence that a woman in possession of a La Perla bra and knicker set is far sassier in pursuit of a handsome man than a woman wearing her grey holey period knickers.

Pace Yourself

Bringing Mr Right to heel and getting him to stay there and stop sniffing other bottoms is a serious occupation. You need to devote as much solid effort to it as if it were a work project. However, some days and nights you are not going to feel capable of dolling up and hauling yourself across town to a sticky room full of intimidating strangers, homing in on the one you like the look of, prising him away from ten rapt supermodels with your sensational conversation and knee-trembling looks, and whisking him off. On such occasions – so long as they don't occur every night – give yourself a break. Take time out. (And that's not counting the time you spend footling around at your friends' houses or doing your own thing.)

Devote, say, three nights a week to man hunting. That's enough otherwise you'll become jaded. Sometimes you'd rather sit at home in your dressing gown eating biscuits and watching TV while reading a trashy book – or indeed Dostoyevsky – with a cat on your lap (just because you're a single woman doesn't mean you have to be a total cliché). The trick is to avoid falling into the trap – as comedian Rob Newman once pointed out – of thinking of yourself on your golden wedding anniversary saying to your beloved – and I paraphrase – 'and just think, if I hadn't decided to go to that stinky hot stuffy club at 1am when I was dog-tired instead of creeping home to my nice warm cosy bed we never would have met.' Thinking such thoughts in moderation is alright because it stops the faint-hearted from going into permanent hibernation and prevents the lazy from actually welding their butts to the sofa. But. It is too easy to whip yourself into such a frenzy of guilt and 'What ifs' that you spend every night at a smelly club staring wild-eyed into the dry ice in the vain hope that Mr Right will emerge from it. This does you no good at all because:

A) you become despondent
B) you become exhausted
C) you look exhausted and despondent which isn't greatly alluring.

Be a 1.15am Woman

Men can be sods. If there is plenty of, as they in their arrogance perceive it, 'choice' they will be reluctant to pair up. They reckon they'll wait until Elle McPherson walks in. Which means they rarely like to commit themselves to one woman early on in the evening. Hence you can easily waste four hours of your time and leave early in exasperation. Not so fast. When it's thirty minutes until booting out time, the hounds realize as one man their ambition was greater than their sex appeal and start running frantically around trying to find a woman, any woman to call their own (or at least to parade in front of their sad friends and try and get a snog out of). At this stage, there's no denying that Mr Right doesn't exactly sound like a catch.

However. Until he meets Ms Right, Mr Right isn't a catch. Most men — until their dream woman gives them the eye — are scoundrels. The idea is, he meets you and suddenly he doesn't need to frequent The Blackpool Ritzy in a snuffling pack, he stops not phoning when he said he would, and he never plays horizontal wrestling without ensuring that madam is bouncing off the ceiling with pleasure too. It's common enough for a man — or a woman —

to have a series of nasty, brutish and short relationships, despair of ever being compatible with anyone, even a ginger tabby, then suddenly, inexplicably chance upon the person who wipes the sadness of that miserable, mismatched track record with one slow smile and whispered husk of 'I'm scared because it's never felt like this before.'

Even so, when on the prowl at 1.15am, common sense will tell you to avoid the guy trying to impress the ladies by mooning with a rose clenched between his hairy butt cheeks. The pro of this plan is, you and your hunting partner spend a delightful evening somewhere comfortable – say, your lounge – then zip to the nearest target area (possibly in two cars?) at the witching hour, then make a grand entrance. By this point – and no disrespect to all the women who've hung in there grimly all night – everyone else will be sweaty, bored, and dishevelled. You, in contrast, will be cool, fresh, and gorgeous.

It's Unlikely he's from Mars

Chances are he's an earthling, same as you. So treat him like one. Which means you don't have to amend your way of communicating – well, only slightly. So, should you say something daft, you don't have to sit there thinking 'Oh no, why did I say that, aaawwww wwhyyy – oh what must he think of me?' If you say nothing and retreat into your embarrassment he may think badly of you. Whereas if you say, 'Sorry – I didn't mean you to think I …' etc., he will very probably take pity on you and forgive you.

Real Life, Real Booboo

Lucy, 27: 'The first time I met my now fiancé, at a party, I made a derogatory joke about two women sitting across the room. I thought they'd been looking at us oddly, so I said "They're probably lesbians." It was a foolish glib thing to say and if a man had said it I'd have got defensive (just because two women aren't falling all over you and so what if they are etc.), but anyway, I said it. He replied, in a neutral tone, "My sister's a lesbian." I felt so ashamed I could barely speak. I thought serves you right. Now you've blown it. I could feel my face turning red. I forced myself to look him in the eye and I said "I'm so sorry – that was a terrible thing to say." I couldn't stop myself from adding glumly "I might as well go home now." He burst out laughing. A few months on I asked him what he thought when I made the comment. "I thought, oh," he replied. "But you were so remorseful, I thought Ah well, she's alright."'

First Organized Date

It's practically *official* (that he fancies you). With this comforting knowledge in your head, all you have to do is to confirm it in *his* head. If you don't act smug, say anything wildly offensive or do anything nasty or dastardly, this shouldn't be a problem. Following are a few tips to jog true lust along.

Getting Closer

If you can swing it, arrange to meet somewhere extremely crowded, such as one of those pubs stuffed wall to wall, where everyone jostles and glares and spills their drinks on other peoples' shoulders. Why? Because although these are highly irritating unromantic places, you will be forced into close bodily contact. For a start, everyone has a square inch to themselves so you will have to stand practically pressing against each other. This can add a certain frisson. There are hoards of opportunities, for example some ox pushes past you carrying 20 pints – the dream man is obliged to put a protective arm around your back to push you out of harm's way. Or, some twit barges into you from behind, practically catapulting you into Mr Right's manly chest. For effect, you can press a hand up against it (his chest, for now) to regain your balance.

Jumping the Gun

Assuming all has gone to plan and he is gagging to marry you – joke, sorry – to ravish you, don't ever make the mistake of thinking 'No, no, I needn't shave my legs because I will absolutely not sleep with him until the 15th date' or 'I am going to wear my grey period knickers because that will ensure I don't sleep with him tonight.' Because you may (as you realize he kisses like a god and merely feeling his arms around you makes you want to rip off his clothes and pin him to the floor) change your mind suddenly, then be faced with the bittersweet realization that he is going to try to remove your grey period knickers with his teeth. In all honesty, by this stage, he wouldn't really care if you were wearing purple pantaloons.

However, being a great seductress is a state of mind as much as anything else, and if you feel uncomfortable your mood will communicate itself to him and kill the atmosphere stone dead. From the minute you decide you want him, start preparing yourself. This means total deforestation – under arms, legs, bikini line and, when you have a bikini line wax, don't be shy, demand as much off as you want – any stray hairs on your bottom – order her to whip them off. No one's pretending it's dignified but better your beautician thinks 'My, this woman's hairy'* than the dream man. (Although if he did, and worse, mentioned it, you would be justified in dumping him forthwith – shallow git.) Other precautions: don't wear tights. Just don't. They have horrible gussets and are about as sexy as a bin full of maggots. Men hate them, and any enjoyment of getting it on with the man you lust after is practically ruined by you thinking 'He's going to see my heavy duty tights.'

Trouble is, the alternative is stockings – and although stockings are sexy, they also scream 'I've made the biggest effort in the world, I've trussed myself up like a chicken and worn these just for you'. At this, the game-playing stage, you don't want him to think this is the norm – unless you don't have a job you won't have time to wear stockings every day. You want him to think of stockings as an occasional bonus. Seduction doesn't stop after you've got his boxers off. It should continue for as long as the relationship lasts. Some women avoid the tights/stockings dilemma by wearing trousers or going bare-legged – fine if you are dark-skinned or have a tan (or fake stuff that doesn't turn you orange) – not so fine if you have legs like Roquefort cheese.**

* Don't delude yourself you're any hairier than the rest of womankind – the majority of us are reasonably furry, it's normal.

** If it's a tights-or-nothing situation, wear the horrid things, but if he starts fumbling in the gusset area your best bet is to curl down and peel them off before he registers. You will of course, have taken off your shoes first. I'd practise this manoeuvre in the privacy of your bathroom until you have it down to a slinky art.

Real Seduction, Real Nightmare

Elizabeth, 25: 'I was at college. It was the end of term ball. I knew exactly who I wanted to seduce and exactly what I was going to wear to do it. I invited this guy Gareth – I was friendly with the group of guys he lived with but it was quite a statement to have invited him. He was lovely about it – he sent me a bouquet of red roses before the ball, the first flowers I'd ever received from a man. I had bought a long black clingy dress but the only problem was, my stomach bulged. So I went to Marks & Spencer and bought really big granny pants to squash it in. Elasticized tummy panel, up to the waist, beige hue, the works. All went as planned, the snogging, the groping, and it was only when he slid his hand up my dress when I realized – the pants! He was such a sweet guy I'm sure he wouldn't have cared but I cared. I couldn't stand him to know I was dressed in Victorian pants. I pushed his hands away. Actually, it worked out. He realized nothing was going to happen that night, and very sweetly kissed me goodbye at my door. We got it together a few days later. I was wearing my sexiest flimsiest pants, if you must know.'

The Champagne Kiss

It's such a cute little trick. You finally kiss, bells ring, birds sing, it's all glorious, he doesn't slobber like a Bloodhound or have a tongue like an old slab of plaice. You go on kissing for some time. Then you introduce some champagne into the equation. You take a gulp of cold champagne, French kiss him and squirt some of the liquid into his mouth so it fizzles, bursts, and tingles – don't squirt too hard or he may choke. It's an unexpected tingly pleasure, suggests to him you're a woman of many talents, and makes him shiver from his cute head to his smallest toes.

Swot Note

Your kisses should hold promise. If you're kissing standing up, arch against him and don't be afraid to rub up a little. Put one hand on the back of his head and the other on the small of his back. Julie, 24, says, 'I was kissing my boyfriend at a party and his friend Luke said I looked as if I was worshipping him with my body. I reckon that's a good thing.' A sexy little trick is to kiss and suck his upper lip (not exclusively) because apparently, its effects go straight to the groin.

Alluring Date Protocol

You're going out to eat – or rather, he is taking you out to eat.

A) If he asks you to suggest a venue, don't say 'I don't mind.' It's polite, but boy is it tiresome. Most men, if they're keen, will have a few ideas about where they want to take you (begins with b and ends with d and has an e in the middle). But if he asks for your opinion, have an opinion – it is allowed. If you can't think of anywhere conducive to reeling him in, say 'I do know a place but I can't remember what it's called – I'll find out and ring you back' – then ask your friends to recommend the funkiest/most atmospheric/most fun place they can think of. Tried and tested is best. Don't rely on reviews – better to ask the opinions of people who know what you like. It's best not to choose somewhere impossibly posh and 'romantic' – the contrived atmosphere is pressurizing at the least, excruciating at the most. It makes both of you uncomfortably self-conscious, and dammit, you don't want to be on your best behaviour. Better somewhere loud, reasonably raucous, where you can relax, enjoy yourselves, laugh loudly without the entire restaurant turning to stare, and get into a juicy conversation without being bothered by the waiter sweeping the table with a silly little brush.

B) The Food: eat. Normal men like a woman with a healthy appetite. A woman who eats like an anorexic sparrow, who picks at her mixed salad (no dressing) like it's poisoned, refuses dessert and pats her flat as an ironing board stomach and says 'Phew I'm stuffed' is – as far as her date can see – a liar, liar, pants on fire. Women who see virtue in starving themselves may, occasionally, stoke a man's paternal instinct – he'll want to feed you up and protect you because you're obviously such a damn fool you won't eat enough without being nagged. But men who are very attracted by a woman who starves herself (entirely different, of course, to a woman who is naturally skinny) are, to be frank, odd. An attitude like that betrays a curious view of women – as if he thinks they should be small and weak. A man who feels distaste for a woman who can eat two Big Macs then say 'Where's the apple pie?' has problems.

I'll jump to the conclusion that he is threatened by strong women. Which is to say, a good, sexy man – a man worth seducing – is far more likely to go for you if you eat like a normal human being. Think *Nine and a Half Weeks*. Food is sexy, watching a woman eat is sexy.

This isn't to say you should order everything on the menu to the point where you feel nauseous and your trouser button pops. But have fun with your food.

C) Order something sexy. You can either be brazen and order oysters – hmm – possibly too blatant, but if you are flirting outrageously at this stage go for it. You don't, however, want him to think you're snarfing as many extortionate delicacies as you can stuff at his expense, so say something like 'We'll go halves' – a nicely ambiguous statement. Mussels (used by editors everywhere to illustrate features on the vagina) are, providing they're fresh, less expensive and less obvi- ous, but just as saucy. The idea is to get him thinking about sex any which devious way you can. Spaghetti is good because it's slithery and you can suck it up (he may think 'blow job') – although admittedly, if you splatter tomato sauce all over your face and top at the same time he may just think 'messy eater.' To be on the safe side, choose a spaghetti dish with lemon and butter and herbs so if it does splatter a little, it won't make you look like he can't take you anywhere.

D) Pinching food off his plate: cute, but not that cute. If you ask him for a chip, there's his cue to feed you one. But don't hint: 'Ooh, those chips look nice, I wish I'd ordered some,' and grab a bunch off his plate. Men are territorial about their food. They don't like people pinching it. Also, he probably has a back catalogue of ex-girlfriends who never ordered their own dessert then scooped up two-thirds of his so fast their arms nearly popped out of their sockets – i.e. it conjures up bad memories – he wishes you'd just order your own, and it frustrates him that you didn't. He doesn't understand that some women feel the calories don't count if they come off someone else's plate. And even if he did, he'd just think 'that's daft.' Yet, you can have fun with each other's food. Ask him if he wants to taste yours (rude pun intended, see below) and if he does and then hesitates, scoop up a little on your fork and feed it to him. If he scoops up some of your food with his own fork, or looks as if he is about to, he's missed (you judge whether accidentally or not) a supreme flirting opportunity and can best be described as a goober.

Real Life, Real Sauce

Laura, 26: 'I remember being in McDonalds when I was 11. There was a man and a woman eating Filet o' Fish burgers at the table next to us. The man had spilt some mayonnaise on the side of his mouth, and the woman reached out, scooped it up with her finger and sucked the mayonnaise off her finger. At that age, I thought it was a disgusting thing to do. Now, I think it was an erotic thing to do.'

Don't Swan Off Early

Unless you can't stand him. Otherwise, however valid your reason he'll think it's an excuse. He'll assume you loathed him and will never call you again. (Unless you've struck lucky with a man who knows it's destiny from the second he spied you – but, sigh, that's relatively rare.) Even if you have the most important job interview of your little life in the morning – tough. You are just going to have to survive on adrenaline. Organize your diary better or shake off the shackles of your primary school headmistress and learn to wing it occasionally. Everyone else does, why do you have to be the prissy miss?

Putting Thoughts into his Head

You can do this by innuendo, what you wear, or what you do. For example if you've invited him over, one little ploy is to have your prettiest, laciest knickers and bra drying elegantly in the bathroom. Don't go through the entire chore of wearing them and washing them – take them straight out of your underwear drawer, and cutely arrange them on the washing line or radiator. When he goes to the toilet he will see them and a chain of evil thoughts will begin (if it hasn't already) in his head. He'll think about you in them, you out of them, him peeling them off you, you modelling them for him, what happens after you model them for him. It's not exactly a strain to get him to think about sex with you.

You can also use words with double meanings. As long as you don't become a scary one-woman pastiche of *The Benny Hill Show*, talking about sex – whether frankly or inadvertently – with a gorgeous woman is almost as exciting to a man as doing it.

A Dash of Rejection

Of course you want to play games – what else is seduction about? Indeed, it would be pretty charmless if you didn't dance around each other a little. You shouldn't be too eager because plain willingness, optimism, and openness at the start of a potential relationship are often meanly interpreted by men as desperation. Infuriatingly, they can be as easily put off by a woman who plays it cool. Men are stubborn with delicate egos, and they hate being rejected. Be very, very careful when playing coy because it can backfire. Don't over-analyse and punish him with coolness because of a perceived slight. (You think it's rude not to call within three days, he called on the fourth.) Make allowances for his way of operating.

Real Life, Real Disaster

Jayne, 28: 'I once messed up a blossoming relationship because I acted like I felt I should, rather than how I wanted to. We were just getting to know each other. We'd been out to dinner once, he'd given me a chaste kiss goodbye in the taxi, then I'd been over to his place where he'd cooked me dinner and he'd talked and kissed a little more. Then,

I invited him over to me for dinner (it was quite dinner oriented) for the Friday of the following week. If I'd been him, I would have called the day before to confirm the date was still on and to check what time I was expected. But he didn't call until two hours before he was actually due at my house. By that time, I'd convinced myself he wasn't going to turn up. So when he said "Is it still on?" I pretended – in a mad attempt to be cool – that I'd forgotten and was now busy. His voice went cold, and when I said "But can we do it another time?" he said "Sure" and rang off. I did phone him again but he was always "busy." I got the message. It was my own fault for trying to be too clever.'

Try Anything Once

(And if it doesn't work, quell your mortification by laughing about it later with friends.) What the hell. Say you're having a great 24 hours. You're kicking butt at work, your friends and parents adore you, you're having a sensational hair day, you feel gorgeous inside and out, and you have just made an expensive yet frivolous purchase and you're glad glad glad about it – in fact you're busting all over with self-esteem and other goodies and you can probably get away with anything. Strike while you're feeling hot!

That said, nothing can prick your pink balloon of complacency like a cool snub from an unreceptive man (whose fiancée is standing next to him only you didn't realize). So it would help if you give his body language a quick going over (it's mostly obvious but briefly: twitching, tense jaw, shiftiness, fidgeting, crossed arms, stepping back, no eye contact, ball and chain – all bad news) and do a swift spot check for glowering girlfriends. If he tests negative for both of the above, pick the approach that suits your character best:

- the bop-him-on-head-with-club approach
- the I'll-sizzle-you-simmer, or

- the Holly Golightly facade (perfectly poised but not really).

Just ensure you don't bottle out and start flubbering. Let us take four random situations and knock his prim probably from Next little socks off:

Situation: you're introduced to a bodacious man.

- Zzzt!: 'Hello. And don't you look good enough to eat.' (smirk).
- Cool as: 'Hi. How's it going?' (Let him see you look him up and down.)
- Perfectly poised: 'Enchanted!' (Please purr this word.)
- Rubbish: imperceptible nod as too shy to catch his eye.

Situation: he makes a reference to 'your boyfriend' to see if you have one:

- Zzzt!: 'Actually darling, that situation's vacant' (think: rrrraow!)
- Cool as: 'I don't have a boyfriend. They're not compulsory, you know.' (coyly).
- Perfectly poised: 'And what boyfriend might that be?' (suppressed grin).
- Rubbish: 'Oh! I'm not going out with anyone at the moment. We split up you see.' (Silly, Miss Marpleish worried face, keen to explain).

Situation: end of first meeting:

- Zzzt!: 'You'll be hearing from me.' (Wink, if you absolutely must).
- Cool as: 'Give me a ring, if you like.' (Ditto).
- Perfectly poised. 'I shall await your call.' (Ditto.)
- Rubbish: 'Do you want my number? My work number...my home...my e-mail...mobile...pager...but I'll be at my mother's tomorrow night and that's...'

Situation: you've just kissed properly:

- Zzzt!: 'Oh Maverick, you big stud!' (ott hair-flick)
- Cool as: 'Remind me how you did that again...' (coy is my middle name.)
- Perfectly poised: (smouldering smile.)
- Rubbish: 'I think you're giving me stubble rash. Never mind.' (slight peeved look.)

NB If this is the case, don't bleat. Make him shave – or shave him yourself. This may sound draconion but if you suffer in silence, you will awake the following morning with a large ugly disfiguring raw patch on your chin which will get infected and ooze yellow puss – or, if you're lucky – dry out into a huge purple scab, meaning that if he wants to see you again in the near future you'll have to regretfully turn him down, or grin and vainly attempt to disguise it under a slather of cover up cream. At this stage you want

him to think of you as more beauteous than Marilyn
Monroe, Raquel Welch, and Nikki Taylor squidged into
one. A large scab, sadly, will foil your plan.

Shameless Behaviour

Again, only for restricted use, best employed when feeling confident and the mood calls for exaggerated measures, for example:

- smoking a big fat phallic cigar
- sucking on an ice cube then crunching it
- pouting
- scooping a dollop of cream off the top of his or your Guinness and licking it off your finger
- pinching his bottom (never in the US)
- twirling your hair or twirling his hair
- speaking in deep husk.*

---

* All of the above are enormous fun but run the risk of him calling your bluff. In one husking instance, the target boldly enquired 'Why are you whispering? Is there something wrong with your voice?' The rat.

Never Panic Pre-Date

Eight am. You know what you want to wear tonight. Your black boots, your grey v-neck sweater, and your black trousers. You look great in your black trousers, mostly. You are meeting him straight from work – and you refuse to wear your work clothes – so you're going to change into your sexy kit in the Ladies. You bring the boots, v-neck, and trousers neatly folded in a bag. Excellent – you're all set. Twelve am, and you start thinking about your black trousers. Sometimes they crease around the crotch and you hate that. You decide, at lunch time, just quickly, to have a dress rehearsal. Can't do any harm. My god, what the hell do you look like? The trousers look awful! Have the trousers shrunk? Have you grown? Why did you choose these trousers? You can't stand these trousers. You can't possibly wear them tonight! What were you thinking? Your heart pounding, you scrabble out of the trousers, yank on your work clothes, furiously scrumple the trousers into a bag, throw the bag under your desk and rush out into the street. The only shops within running distance – and you only have 30 minutes – are Marks & Spencer and Next. They'll have to do. You plunge into the throng, barging past other shoppers, out of my way, out of my way, trying to scan the floor in one all-seeing 365 degree sweep. Black, forget it, purple, are you kidding, yellow, no way actually ... yellow. Yellow? Yellow trousers! Bright, beautiful sunshiney yellow, bright trousers, bright personality – you lunge for them, yes! Your size! You grip the hanger and queue impatiently for the changing room, wriggle into them, you're sweaty, rushed, panicked, but yes, they'll do. What about a top to match? You haven't time to try it on, so you grab the yellow jumper in your size. You pay, and ten minutes and eighty quid later, you're home, safe, sitting at your desk. Two pm. The green bag rests at your feet, the adrenaline is still pumping, you feel exhausted but triumphant. The afternoon ticks slowly by – and tonight you're doing no one any favours. Six pm. On the dot. You switch off your computer and glide to the Ladies. You throw off your suit, open your Marks & Spencer bag, bite off the plastic thingies that attach the clothes' label to the price instead of using scissors, nearly pulling out a tooth, and eagerly slink in to your new purchases.

Which is exactly how you end up meeting your date looking like a banana.

Damage Limitation

(If you had too much to drink and made a great trolloping fool of yourself.)

Reasons to be Reassured

If he is as ratted as you are, it won't matter. He will simply think that your trick of eating peanuts from his crotch, or your jape of jumping on to that silver XJS and bouncing on the roof, or the way you ran off with a traffic cone on your head and _____ (fill in your own cringey scenario here) is the most entertaining action he has ever seen in his life bar *Die Hard With A Vengeance*, and what a fun woman you are to be around. (Anyway, like you should worry – you weren't the one stomping along the road roaring at lamp posts 'Come and have a go if you think you're hard enough.') Even if he wasn't legless, unless he's a romantic man or a tad conservative man (in which case he may very probably be appalled and wonder if you're an alcoholic), as long as it doesn't happen every time he sees you (the novelty may wear thin) he may be, I kid you not, although I am trying to be kind – charmed. Admittedly, charmed is a strange word to use – especially if he is holding your hair off your face as you vomit copiously in a corner of the street. Yet, when you are disgracefully drunk, you tend to reveal the less inhibited you – and certainly, if this means starting fights with waitresses and mooning at the opera, stick to orange juice. But, if you merely become loud, raucous, and a tad obnoxious, he may (the patronizing sod) think it's cute. It may reinforce his outrageous male stereotyping, namely that women can't hold their drink. What do you care, so long as it gets you off the hook?

He'll also think you need him to protect you as you're temporarily vulnerable – and men do like to indulge in a bit of Tarzanish chest-beating, so all is not lost.

This is, after all, the *Loaded* generation, and men are used to and revel in bad behaviour. They also like to know that a gorgeous, intelligent, sophisticated woman isn't above a bit of vomiting in the street herself.* It makes them think they can have it all – it makes them think, 'Haha, if I was to take it further with this woman, she'd be relaxed, she'd understand me, she wouldn't nag me for getting ratted with my pals and forgetting to call'. Well – ho ho ho – let him dream. He's not to know that what's sauce for the goose isn't sauce for the gander and, furthermore, should the gander get sauced, he's going to cop it regardless of the goose's own sauce habits.

---

* As long as it's an occasion rather than the norm.

If you think you were severely out of order at any point (we're talking projectile vomit down his Paul Smith shirt and possibly a splatter on his chin), and through your blurry haze you see naked distaste in his eyes (come on, be fair to the poor guy), then a grand gesture may be required. Maybe a new shirt, maybe a bouquet. Men hardly ever receive flowers, but provided the blooms aren't delivered to the rugby club, they are just as much suckers for foliage as women are. It reduces them to blushing, chuffed mumblers. And for those sensitive types, good florists can put together a very macho clutch of blooms – full of twigs, thorns, and big leaves. The note should read something like 'Oops, sorry.' Even the uptight romantic man can be pacified this way (Paul Smith shirts are washable, and my goodness it was gross but it's not as if you spat at his mother*) If he's worth the angst he should calm down and give you another chance.

Worst Case Scenario

Carla, 27: 'I was just getting it together with this guy. A friend was having a drinks party and I invited Pete. He had a dinner to attend but said he'd turn up later. I don't drink much at all, never have done. But that night I was so nervous, I started knocking back neat tequila – I hated the taste but kept going. By the time Pete arrived I was semi-comatose. At one point, my friends called a taxi to take me

* If you did, maybe you'll have to let this one go.

to hospital to have my stomach pumped, but the driver wouldn't let me get in. All I remember is Pete giving me a fireman's lift up to his room – it was the first time his flatmates had met me so it wasn't a great first impression. I think I must have hurled at some point because I woke up in Pete's bed feeling fine. He was sitting fully clothed in the middle of the room. He'd watched me all night to make sure I didn't expire. It wasn't my ideal seduction plan, especially the weeing bit. To his credit, I think he was only mildly horrified. Possibly he thought he'd seen me at my worst, so it could only get better.'

He Pays and Other Old-Fashioned Rules

If he asks you out on a first date, courtesy demands that he pays. Nothing to do with sexism – it's the same if you ask a client to join you for lunch, you pay. (Of course, if you ask your mother to join you for coffee, she pays – but she's the exception that proves the rule.) However. It is not nice to assume. You are a modern, independent woman, not a spoiled brat, and courtesy also demands that you offer to pay. You don't have to offer to pay the entire bill – although if it's been a blast, why not – but he'll appreciate it if you suggest making a contribution. As he gets out his plastic, reach for your bag and say 'Let me help you with that.' This is the test. Either he says:

■ 'Absolutely not! How dare you! Put that away!' (Steady dear, it's a purse not a gun. Suggests he's a tad conservative and thinks ladies should never pay for their own dinners. A double-edged sword, this one, because he'll also think, I'll be bound, that ladies should have long shiny hair down to their bottoms.)

- 'No please, let me.' (Polite, well-mannered, but no indication of whether he feels pleased or merely obliged.)
- 'This is my shout! You can pay next time.' (Healthy, sweet-natured man! Also telling you quite plainly he's keen to meet up again. Excellent, meriting a gold star.)
- 'Are you sure? Well, if you insist.' (Cheapskate.)

Or he totes up the bill, working out precisely what you both owe. (Pay what you owe, then bid him a cold goodnight and never see him again.)

What Now?

If he flips when you offer to help pay, the sweet thing to do is to say 'Are you sure? Well thank you very much.'

If he coolly insists on paying, the sweet thing to do is to say 'Are you sure? Well thank you very much.' There's no need to launch into a great palaver of 'Are you sure you're sure ... no really ... are you really sure bore bore.' He's said he'd like to pay, you questioned him once, he's reassured you, fine. That's it. You'll take his word for it, you're both adults conversing like adults, you'll believe him – you haven't got time to play word games all night.

Annoyance Note

However. It has been known for a man to respond at this point 'You didn't put up much of a fight!' To which you archly reply: 'Was I supposed to?'

If he suggests that you pay next time – assuming you want there to be a next time – you treat him to your most devastating smile and say 'Thank you very much. I will pay next time.' Thus, you graciously accept and you let him know you too are keen to meet up again.

If he lets you pay half, either he is desperately desperately short of cash or – and this is more probable – he isn't as mad keen as we thought. He's also mildly rude. Let it pass, but to be frank, it doesn't bode brilliantly. If he totals up exactly what you owe, write him off. Now.

Charisma and How to Acquire it

Hard, but let's work on it. Unfairly, charisma tends to be something you either have or you don't. People who aren't born with it but ape it are often described as 'wacky,' and that's by their friends. Happily, charisma takes many different forms and rarely involves wearing brightly coloured hats. If you try to be charismatic by acting in a way that truly isn't you, others tend to see through it and mentally put you down as insecure. It makes them edgy and wary of you because if you're putting on an act you're patently not a relaxed or relaxing person. The dictionary definition of charisma is: 'A special personal quality or power of an individual making him' (and her – bloody cheek) 'capable of influencing or inspiring large numbers of people.' So, practically any trait that makes other people warm to you, want to be like you or feel great about themselves, for instance:

- The ability to make other people scream with laughter.
- An unquenchable enthusiasm and energy for life.
- A free spirit.
- Personal strength tempered with vulnerability.

- Confidence, optimism and self-sufficiency.
- Unaffected eccentricity.
- Passion.
- Generous intelligence.

Thing is, if you try to play upon any of these assets, they lose their charm. It's easier to be aware of uncharismatic traits and try to underplay them, for example:

- pessimism
- apathy
- dependency
- blatant weakness
- insecurity
- affected eccentricity
- patronizing intelligence.

You don't have to be smart to realize that a happy, amusing, sparky, original self-confident person is delightful to be around whereas a miserable, clingy, whingebag is not.

Let him See You in your Field of Expertise

A great many people fall in love at work, partly because it's convenient, but also because if you are attracted to a person, it is extremely arousing to watch them be clever at something. You witness him dealing competently with a client and – probably because you feel deprived of attention and turned on by his power and professionalism – you want to tear off his clothes and ravish him on the desk. He'll feel the same about you. If, until now, he has only seen the social you, treat him to a glimpse of the formal you – even if that means he meets you outside your office and you trot out deep in serious conversation with a be-suited colleague. Ideally, you'd like him to see you in full flow – and if you work in an unstuffy environment maybe he can be shown up to your office? Promise him you'll be five minutes, and make sure it's not a second more or he'll stop being impressed and start feeling as if he's being made to hang around for hours while you show off.

Quick One: Flexibility

One only has to be in the gym dutifully puffing away on the exercise bike when a madam who does yoga swans in and starts performing contortionist-like exercises in front of the mirror to know that men are mightily impressed by a bendy woman. They drool like puppies. They are, of course, imagining her performing all these elaborate leg-over-head manoeuvres in the bedroom. If you are double-jointed and can do the splits, join a gym immediately and start making heads turn.

The Last Minute Invitation: What to Do

Depends what stage the seduction is at. If this is the first time he has called after your first ever meeting – say, three days later he calls you at work – 'How are you ... yeah, ah, I wondered if you were free tonight – I've got tickets to this play/gig/match.' My dear, unless it is your mother's birthday, you say YES. You say yes because although we could assume he's already asked six other women and you're the last-ditch seventh choice, we could equally assume that he wants to ask you out but is nervous of rejection and needs an excuse to ask you (hence – the tickets flew onto his desk, out of thin air, and suddenly he needs someone to help him use them up). In his mind, if he were to ask you out today for Saturday night the stakes are high – it's a big boogie night, he is putting his ego on the line, revealing he has nothing to do other than take you out.

This way (the tickets tonight way), it's much more casual. This is the last-minute invitation to say yes to, because if you reject the first invitation, unless he is one of those ghastly men who won't take 'No I'm busy for the next 60 years but please, try me then' as a No, he won't ask you again. The ones you really want rarely do. So, you go. You give him the benefit of the doubt. Next time, it's a no. No you are not bloody available to go out with him on Saturday night when he calls at 4.30pm the same day. What – does he think you're grizzling around in leggings waiting for his call? No need to answer that one – it was a rhetorical question. You are, of course, gracious: 'I'd love to, Mark/Michael/John – but I'm busy.'

You don't explain. Let him think that one of the Armani models (the one with a degree) is jetting you to Paris for the evening. No need to let on it's your Aunt Maureen's silver wedding anniversary and the whole family is going on a jaunt to Garfunkels. If you must, add 'Why don't we speak next week, maybe we can arrange something for next weekend?' Thus you don't put him off too sharply but – without being explicit – you let him know that if he requires the pleasure of your company he'll have to – pardon the expression – get his arse in gear.

If the First Date is Awful

Many a first date is disastrous – and the two of you still end up married (to each other). Try to distinguish between nerves and ghastly personality. Sometimes your intuition can tell you that beneath this showoffy loudmouth is a healthily insecure guy with real generosity of spirit. Or maybe those awkward pauses are because he's in awe and a little tongue-tied – not because he's a bore or has nothing to say to you. Then he's worth a second chance.

Not Worth a Second Chance

Lara, 24: 'I'm Jewish and when I mentioned this to my date he said in surprise "But you've got a small nose – did you have a nose job?"!! I said, "Yeah, and I had my horns shaved off too." It was stupidity rather than hatred, but I don't think stupidity excuses prejudice, and the second he said it I knew I had no future with this person. However kind, sexy, and funny he might turn out to be, he had alienated me at a fundamental level. No doubt he also thought all Scots were penny-pinching and all Afro-Caribbeans had great rhythm.'

Worth a Second Chance

Grace, 29: 'Four years ago, I went on a blind date with this guy which was set up through a friend of mine. He insisted on picking me up – and he was an hour late. By this time I'd given up on him and was settled in front of the TV eating crisps. When he rang the doorbell I was furious – he looked lovely and I stank of cheese and onion. He was very apologetic – he'd got a flat tyre and he hadn't known how to fix it and he'd left my number at home. This made me think 'Pathetic!' I was in a very bad mood. When we got to the restaurant we were so late, they'd given away our table. He was laid back, which infuriated me further. We ended up in a chippy and I had to grudgingly admit it was fun, but when we returned to his car someone had, unfortunately, sprayed paint on it. He was gutted. He was so upset. I said rudely, 'It's not as if someone ran over your dog', and he said 'No, but it's my mother's car.' He dropped me home and I didn't invite him in, the mummy's boy! I rang my best friend immediately to sound off. She listened, then said quietly 'Actually Grace, he sounds very sweet – his only crimes are being easy-going, wanting to impress you, and knowing sod all about cars.' I have to say, four years on, he is still easy going, wants to impress me, and knows sod all about cars – and I really don't mind.'

Distinguish between:

- rudeness/being direct
- pomposity/wanting to share some information

- sarcasm/teasing
- reputation/fact
- boasting/enthusiasm
- being aloof/shyness
- formality/terror of offending you
- boredom/nervous paralysis
- immaturity/playfulness
- vanity/making an effort
- naivety/stupidity.

The Ringing Game

There are best possible scenarios for different personalities.

If you cannot resist temptation, the bps is that he has taken your number and you don't have his, or indeed, any way of getting it. This means you are not tempted to ring him the same evening 'Just to check you got home safely' or any other piddly pathetic I'm desperate reason. It also means you are at liberty to continue living your life, (going out, socializing, walking the dog, working, shopping etc.,) as it was before you met him. You are also, unfortunately, at liberty to stay in, for the forseeable future, intermittently picking up the receiver to see if it works and if your mother calls dismissing her a tad sooner than is polite saying 'I'm expecting an important call.'

What does the seductive expert do? She goes out and leaves a jaunty message on her answer machine saying 'Hi, I'm out, please leave an exciting message.' She does not leave a message on her answer machine saying 'Hi, I'm out, but I can be contacted at my mother's until 12, on this number, then I'll be on the tube for half an hour but you can leave a message on my mobile, and if you don't want to do that, then after 1pm I'll be in Waitrose but I'll be back here at 2.30'. If he wants to contact you he will. It makes no difference to him if you are in or out – if he wants to get in touch he will leave a message. It is heart-breakingly unfair, but you can't force it. (Well, you can a bit, hence this book.)

If You're the Brooding Type

The bps is that you secure his number. If possible, don't give him your number unless he demands it – otherwise, knowing you, you'll think 'Well if he hasn't called, why should I call him?' Before you know it, you've talked your-self into a huff and out of ever speaking to the poor man again. As we were saying. You secure his number. Then wait five days. If he is truly, cross–your–heart–hope–to–die keen, phone earlier. Two days is a good rule. But if you even suspect he might be the conceited type, do not call until day five. This type benefits from the you-want-can't-have treatment.

You Call Him Protocol

Dial 141 before you call. Then if he isn't home, don't leave a message. Call back later. Be aware that if he dials 1471 the tittle-tattle BT woman is going to tell him the caller withheld their number, and if he has any intuition, he may think it's you. So if he says, 'Did you call earlier?' be prepared to smoothly deny it. If he isn't in again, don't call any more times that day – maybe he's screening his calls, you don't know. The Very Worst Possible Scenario is that he has caller ID. Now that could be embarrassing.

When you speak to him never say 'Why didn't you call?' (These sort of accusations come much, much later in relationships and they aren't seductive then, either).

If your jaunty conversation is wearing thin, end the call. Don't loiter.

If he likes you it won't matter a jot that you called him before he called you. Millions of impatient happily married women are testimony to the fact that phoning him before he phones you isn't the biggest booboo in the world. Furthermore, you cut out five days of sloping around in your pyjamas agonizing.

If you call and it's a disaster. He sounds surprised to hear your voice and says he's 'busy at work' at the moment. This, as we all know, is coward's code for 'I'm not interested.' Fine. You say, 'Sure. Okay, bye.' Then stick your tongue out at the phone to make yourself feel better. Now, you can stop wondering 'Did he lose my number?' because you know he isn't interested. Jump up and down to shake him off. His loss, as we say.

Enthusiasm: Be Full of It

He asks you for a second date. Don't say, oh so casually, because you're so laid back, 'Oh yeah, sure ... I don't think I'm doing anything that night.' Well, he's just put his ego on the line and you've trodden on it. Now, doubtless, he's desperate for your company. No. If you want to up the seduction process a notch, you put a sizeable measure of chuffedness into your voice, and say 'I'd love that!' If you sound less than enthusiastic, he may think 'She's not interested' and backtrack. If he's touchy (not unheard of) he may say, 'Well, don't force yourself. Look, I'll see you around.' Pank! Or, he may just stand you up. Ouch.

When you see him, you are also allowed to say something nice – it's up to you whether you want to be plain complimentary – 'Nice jacket' – more personal – 'cool haircut!' – or seductively purry – 'Mmm, you smell nice.' This may sound too girly, but men grow up in a largely compliment-free zone. Even if his parents did praise him, a man's friends rarely say sweet things to him. If he scores a goal, then yes. If he gets a promotion, then maybe. If he has a nice haircut, very probably no. He may grin and look sheepish but chances are, he is genuinely pleased. Easy.

The Friendly Shoulder Massage

The very friendly shoulder massage. Men – let's not be coy, most of us – associate a massage with sex. Which is why a good friend got in a huff when her mother-in-law organized a massage for said friend's husband for Christmas – 'His own mother!' she squealed in fury. A tad over the top, but you can understand why a woman doesn't leap at the idea of another woman fondling her husband's bare back right down to and including the top of his buttocks. Yes, fondling. A massage is fondling in thin disguise – it's stroking, kneading, sensual touch, which is exactly why you should brush up on your massage skills and when he and you are sitting together in a cosy venue and he confesses he's tense and stressed because work was a nightmare today, you purr 'What you need is a neck massage.'

Better that you are in the near vicinity, for example, he's sitting at your kitchen table, you're behind him making coffee – so you can swizzle round, place your hands gently on his shoulders, and start squeezing and giving him goose pimples as you say 'You need a massage.' If you say 'You need a massage' then get up, scraping your chair, and purposefully plod over, it will look awkward and almost staged as if you plotted it! Ha ha, the very idea. As you knead, pummel and reduce him to jelly, he will be thinking lascivious thoughts – your hands fondling the rest of his body, for instance...

Massage Tips to Jellify

- Always keep at least one hand in contact with his body.
- Keep the movements slow and rhythmic.
- Vary the pressure from light to firm – don't be too vicious.
- If he's a nail man, gently stroke his neck with your fingernails.
- If he receives this treat with enthusiasm, breathe gently on his neck before kissing it, then blow on his skin. He should be good and goosepimply by now.

To Hold Out or Put Out?

Part One

We're not discussing this as a moral issue, it is simply posed in order to determine what will bring Mr Right yapping to heel. Fact is, there are hoards of happily married women – probably the same lot who called too soon – who capitulated on the first date – worse, they made the first move, the hussies! And, by god they've been punished for their harlotry, with their adoring husbands who think they're the most wonderful things since lager was invented ... Here's the truth: if the spark is instant, if you two are so compatible, if you're both free and single, it doesn't matter a bean if you rut like rabbits within five hours of meeting for the first time (sorry, am I being conservative here?). If he likes you and is right for you, he isn't going to think – in that admirably unself-aware way that some men do – she did it with me and we're practically strangers – she's a tart – (me? I'm er, I'm a red blooded heterosexual male etc.). Most men are a little insecure and – later on – he may quiz you as to whether you always sleep with men on the first date. Partly because he's got a nerve. Partly because he wants to reassure himself that he's special.

Possible Answers

- 'Oh yes, always. There's no point in getting to date number twenty then realizing he has a matchstick penis, is there?' (*deadpan*).
- 'Never, if you must know. But (*exaggerated sigh*) you swept me off my feet and out of my knickers.'
- 'Actually, I've never slept with anyone, ever. (*Dramatic pause, plus slightly loony stare*) You're my first. Now ve haf to marry.'*
- 'Why do *you* ask?'
- 'Well, you don't buy a car without test-driving it first.'
- 'No, why – do you always sleep with men on the first date?'

If he is Mr Right, he'll understand what you're saying.

Part Two

However, here are some reasons you might want to keep your knickers on:

If you don't have sex, you suspect you'll never see him again. If this is the feeling you get from him, have no doubt: this man is after a one-night stand, and you'll never see him again whether you de-knicker or not. Never do it because you think he expects it. He doesn't expect it. He's just trying it on.

---

* Only if you think he can take it.

Some men prefer to wait. Not because of you. Because of them. Some men have to feel ready. Gee, they're not all always-up-for-it-robots. They get flustered and feel pressured (all the things we delicate flowers are supposed to feel) and embarrassed, and therefore never call you again.

Or they have double standards and they think 'If she's willing to do it with me, she's probably willing to do it with anyone.' Not exactly a watertight theory, but a man who thinks in such a simplistic way probably isn't the sharpest tool in the box – and that's regardless of whether he's a road sweeper, an Oxford graduate, or both. Then, even if he likes you, it may put him off you. He likes you but he can't respect you!!! The hypocrisy is staggering, and frankly, if that's what he's like about sex, he's going to have a whole set of startling opinions about what women should and shouldn't do, none of which you'd want to stay around to experience. A lot of men will not turn down the first opportunity to get laid with a nice girl, yet they laughably think it's not right for a nice girl to get laid with them at the first opportunity (or whatever dreary timescale they judge her by).

Or, they suspect you might be someone special and they're nervous. Recognize hesitance when you see it. If he isn't returning your fulsome embrace with total commitment, or seems a tad limp (and we're referring to the whole of his body here), pull back, look at him and whisper, 'We're speeding!' and give him a gentle kiss and stop. (If that is too abrupt, and further explanation is required, add, 'I need a coffee – want one?') Keep the mood light. Don't apologize. Unless he said 'geroff me!' and you ignored him you haven't done anything wrong. DON'T think 'oh woe! he doesn't fancy me, I've come on like a prostitute, I should be stoned etc.'

Common Sense Note

Don't try to seduce him immediately if the reasoning behind it is 'Sex confirms he likes me.' Sadly, it confirms nothing of the sort. It confirms he fancies you or he fancies a bit and you were willing. It doesn't confirm he wants a relationship. So never do it just because you want reassurance. If you want reassurance, the best way to get it is to go into a small boutique carrying a designer bag, try on an exquisitely expensive dress, and ask the assistant, 'How do I look?'

How to Seduce Your Dream Man

Twelve Point Plan: Awaking the Next Day Looking Ravishing

Last night, you looked ravishing, and it worked. This morning, you look like a puffy toad or, if you're one of the lucky ones, an anaemic panda. He, meanwhile, is sleeping like ... a man. You have six minutes to make yourself look sensational without arousing suspicion:

■ Grab item of clothing – preferably, long sleeved t-shirt (slinky, modest, without bulk). If not, you may have to settle for second best, for example, jumper lying on nearby chair/floor.

■ Find your bag which should always contain cotton bud tips and a small sample tube of moisturizer and rush to bathroom. Splash lukewarm water on face.

■ Remove sleep from eyes.

■ Squeeze tiny dab of moisturizer onto cotton bud and remove smudged mascara. If you don't have any cotton buds fold an edge of toilet paper into a point – any moisturizer will do to remove smudged mascara – and other old make-up.

- Also use moisturizer to moisturize rest of face.
- Pinch your cheeks to make yourself look less sallow.
- Squeeze glob of toothpaste onto finger and vigorously clean teeth (even better if you always carry your own mini-toothbrush – the sort they give you on planes.)
- Find brush and brush hair. If no brush available, finger comb your hair.
- If your eyes are puffy, curl your eyelashes to make your eyes look less like small currants in a bun.
- If your lips are dry, smear dab of Vaseline on them – will give them slight sheen without it being obvious you're cheating.
- Any blemishes – grab cotton bud and cover up, and blend out worst offenders.
- Leave your bag outside the room and slip back into bed, you Aurora you.

The Evening After

It's not so much the morning after – during which any person with half a brain can rustle up an hour of common civility before heading off for work – it's the evening after, when you're tired and reckless, that's dangerous. Then, there may be an urge to ring him and mention the word 'relationship.' Word of doom! In his mind, rather like Arnold Schwarzenegger denying the existence of the toilet in *Kindergarten Cop*, 'Dere *iss* no relationship!' So don't say the word, or anything akin to it like, 'So what happens now?' This question puts every sliver of power into his great clumsy paws. No no no. Even though you had a fantastic time, even though he was an absolute gentleman and you walked to the station together and he kissed you goodbye – don't ask begging questions.

If you feel an uncontrollable urge to make contact that same day, stamp on it. If you know he's going to be out, and your self-control level is zero, leave a message – although many wouldn't – saying 'Just calling to say thanks for last night – bye!' It is tempting to want to speak to him lots, to convince him via every witty immaculate, exchange that you are a gal in a million and should be snapped up without further ado. Don't. In an ideal world, he'd call you that same evening to say 'I want to see you again. Soon. Would you like to go out for dinner?' He may leave it a horrific five or six days, even, gasp, a week, because he doesn't want to appear pushy or there's been a lot of football on. When he does ring, don't act coolly just because you felt he *should* have called earlier. He doesn't owe you anything. Be friendly – not madly hysterical with joy. The passive-aggressive 'I'm angry with you but I'm not going to tell you why, you work it out' ploy is immature and it freaks men out. They hate it. Be normal, be friendly. This way, you betray nothing except the fact you're pleased (nice, moderate feeling) that he called.

Don't Loiter

Unless you're waiting for a bus, loitering of any kind spells indecision, weakness, and in the worst cases, desperation. And if a man thinks you're desperate he'll be out of your life faster than a cheetah in a McLaren F1. Apply it to all situations – such as talking on the phone (better to have a quickish but snappy upbeat conversation than a long one with awkward pauses). Same goes when talking to him at a party. If you feel a restlessness – beat it. You don't have to be dismissive – touch him on the arm, smile, and say 'I'll see you later.' If you feel it would be bizarre and inappropriate to skedaddle without explanation, say 'I'd better find my friend, or she'll think I've abandoned her. (Subtext: I'm loyal, and I'm not so desperate for your company that I'm going to stand here while you fidget.) See you in a bit.' If it feels right, kiss him on the cheek, then turn tail and walk away.

Catching a Rebound Man

Can be very effective. While some rebound men are bitter, miserable, and best avoided, others can be primed for commitment. They have been holed up in a five year relationship which – for whatever reason – wasn't right. They suddenly realize they want to be in a serious relationship – but not that one. Quite often, after bailing out of such a relationship, men bounce into another one and propose within a fortnight. Not because they were desperate to marry just anyone, but because their not-quite-right relationship threw into relief the things they precisely wanted from a relationship. So, if you catch a rebound man at the right time – he may come to heel with very little dragging.

Probability Note

Rebound men tend to be men you've known for a while, primarily because they've just dumped a good friend of yours or they're the best friend of your just ex-boyfriend. Thus, snaring a rebound man can be a tad tricky and – unless you are so convinced he's Mr Right you'd stake your hamster's life on it – a foolish selfish friendship-ending move. In such a situation you are only justified in seducing him if it ends in marriage.

If Possible Note

The best sort of rebound man is a good friend of yours whose newly-ex girlfriend you don't know terribly well. All your loyalty lies with him and – if you have anything to do with it – so does the rest of you. But slowly does it. If you are wise, you have never blabbed out that you had designs on him. This way, he does not see you as a potential – pardon the language – sympathy shag. If there is one certainty in this book it is that the seductress, as far as the seductee is concerned, is never a certainty. You want him to hope – you don't want him to be complacent. So, when he tells you that his girlfriend of five years standing is now history, your first words are not 'At last! You're freee! For meee!' They are: 'Are you okay? What happened? (Make sure you pause long enough between questions to a. breathe and b. let him speak.) Bide your time before exclaiming, 'Shall I come round?'

If you did blab out, in an unguarded moment, that you love him more than life itself, then you have to play the part of the supportive, platonic friend – resisting all his sneaky plays for a lay – for longer. As long as it takes for him to think you must have changed your mind about him. Then...

Making the Transition from Friend to Lover

Admittedly, the mechanics of this are fairly obvious. But way before any hanky panky occurs, you need to make the transition from friend to lover in his head. The most usual way to do this is to play The Sympathetic Friend. It means he's liable to slope round to avail himself of your kindly nature. This gives you ample opportunity to kiss him on the forehead – a well known maternal habit – which tricks him into believing you have no predatorial thoughts. However, the physical contact plants a seductive seed of possibility in his head.

It also allows you to ply him with a little alcohol to loosen his tongue and inhibitions. It allows you to give him a comforting hug (and – despite his self-pity – to be aware of your bosom pressing against his face). Poor you, you soothe, firmly squashing his head to your chest (let him breathe). He'll stop feeling sorry for himself fairly swiftly, but keep acting in order to prolong the bosom-head arrangement.

Even if he doesn't immediately fall on your bosom –

not to worry. Men often lurch towards the woman who listens and soothes – for two reasons:

- He appreciates the emotional support because his male friends are as unlikely to be as soothing as you can pretend to be, even though, contrary to popular belief, men are perfectly capable of confiding in their very closest friends and their very closest friends are perfectly capable of offering some degree of sympathy. Still, chances are he doesn't find his very closest friend that fanciable.
- By listening and soothing, you validate his feelings and puff up his ego. To be honest, playing the Sympathetic Friend can be a chore. It may well involve nodding for three hours while he talks.

How to Speed Matters Along

Dress to kill – think of it as the bespectacled-secretary-to-secret-agent-sex-kitten transformation. You want him to re-programme his idea of you and this means shock therapy. Glam up to the max, in a devastatingly subtle sophisticated way, of course. Give him the sympathetic bosom-press. Squeeze his arms. Rock him a little. You may also, if you wish, suggest a night out to drown his sorrows. Take him to a comedy night (even if it's awful), share a pizza and a bottle of wine, then stagger home together, suggest watching a video – put on something scary – then sit quite close to him on the sofa, not too close at first, then ... either squeal at the terrifying bits and see if he takes this as an excuse to put his arm around you OR pretend to fall asleep and see if he takes this as an excuse to put his arm around you. Do NOT have sex with him while he or you are drunk. It confuses things. If he's going to bonk you, you want him to know exactly what he's doing and who with and that you're not just in the right place at the right time. You want the transition from friend to lover to be on your terms — and your terms should be:

- He realizes he really really likes you while he is stone cold sober.
- He realizes he's liked you for ages but just hasn't realized.
- He realizes he now has to 'persuade' you to think of him in the same way.
- He finally confesses — hey! you're friends! That's the difference! — his feelings.
- You act flattered but question him — is he sure this isn't a rebound thing?
- You say he's thrown you — can you think about it...

The reason you pause for say, a week, before leaping into his arms, is so you can be sure he means it. Even then, the best policy is to leave it a while before you sleep with him — only because a rebound man is looking for reassurance that he's still a stonking great stud and the simplest way he can get it, he thinks, is to bonk someone. You want to be sure he wants you for your wonderful mind, as well as for your wonderful body. Otherwise it will sour your friendship. Curdled milk will have nothing on you two.

A Nose Ahead

That useful institution, The Smell & Taste Treatment and Research Foundation in Chicago has performed some vital studies into what aromas turn men into buckets of lust. The smells they adore include: vanilla, cola, strawberry, butter popcorn, cinnamon buns, doughnuts and lavender. Which leads anyone with a grain of common sense to believe that inviting a man over for a sickly afternoon tea is the way to nab him.

The menu should be as follows:

- Butter popcorn (aperitif).
- Fresh strawberries, vanilla ice cream, cinnamon scones and squirty cream (cream is sexy in its own right so it's not as if we're distracting him here).
- Coke to drink.
- Then – if he has room – sticky jam doughnuts.

NB forget the lavender – it's for old ladies. It possibly only scored in the research because it reminded a few ex-public schoolboys of their nannies. Fact is, this gargantuan tea will win him over for many reasons:

A) The smells.
B) You're spoiling him.
C) It's kiddie food.
D) He'll get a sugar rush and have to find something to do with the energy.

NB2 the Research Foundation also discovered that men loathe the smell of cranberries, baby powder, and – horror – chocolate.

For the cranberries, we can only surmise that cranberries are a beardy-weirdy OTT-PC health food. Political correctness is about as sexy as being slapped round the face with a dead mackerel. So learn to drink Coke instead, and while you're at it, throw out the natural yoghurt too. It frightens men – they think once you're an item you'll force them to eat it too.

Baby powder – no doubt, it only came second to the smell of fresh nappies. Men, unless the child in question is their own, and sometimes even then, associate babies with scary things like never being allowed out of the house to see their pals, being screamed at, no sex ... you get the drift. Don't have baby powder in the house, even if it does stop your skin from chapping after a bath. Learn to dry yourself properly with a towel.

Chocolate – some mistake, surely? But then, men do tend to prefer savoury junk food to sweet junk food. Get your fix while he's not around, or – and this is for when he's truly hooked – suggest you melt it and lick it off him...

Don't Ask Stupid Pointless Questions

Funny how women get the blame for scheming when the average man can be as manipulative as 40 estate agents. However, Mr Right, we trust, isn't like that. So he doesn't appreciate such traits in his girlfriend (reading this book doesn't count). He finds them unsexy, and off-putting. So, if a seductress is brooding over an issue, she never says any of the following:

Q: Was your ex-girlfriend prettier than me?
His ex girlfriend is ex. He is not with her, he is with you. If you keep up the petty I'm-so-insecure questions he will start to wonder why he is with you. Neuroses are not seductive. Don't mention his ex. She is irrelevant. If he mentions her – if he sees her – he had better have a good reason for it. (For example, she is the mother of his children so they need to maintain contact.) But if there is no reason for him to stay in contact with her other than being 'friends', be adult about it. Be specific, ask if you can compromise – out of respect for him, you can't forbid him to

see her. But, you can ask him, out of respect for you, to see her less often. Ask calmly, at a convenient time, explain yourself, don't beg or become hysterical. Now you're cool.

Q: Does this make me look fat?
Oh please. You know he hates this question. He can't win. If you don't like the way it looks, don't wear it. If you feel fat and don't like it, eat less cake.

Q: Am I annoying you?
You may as well add, 'Am I totally pathetic?' The only way this question should ever be asked is if he's done something rude like sigh blatantly while you're talking, or rolled his eyes. Then it should be asked in a sharp, you'd-better-explain-yourself manner.

NB if he does sigh or roll while you're talking, his entitlement to the name of Mr Right is dubious. Discuss (with close female friend).

Q: Don't you fancy me anymore? (Ad nauseam till he runs out the door.)
This, like the three before it, is a dead-end statement. It is hostile, inviting confrontation. You don't really want a serious considered answer (although it would serve you right if he gave you one), you want to provoke him into a disagreement.

Parade Yourself Dripping Wet

- When he's due to pick you up, shower, wash your hair, dress, glam up, but don't dry your hair (unless your wet look resembles a dunked Yorkshire terrier, in which case do the full blow-dry thing a good half hour before he's expected).
- Get caught in the rain.
- Ask him to join you for a swim.

Er, Why Exactly? Note

In formal situations, people tend to be dry. The Cabinet might stretch to calling each other by first names, but is unlikely to assemble in a swimming pool. And, in the initial stages of the seduction – unless you meet on the beach – that's how he'll see you. Dry. Wetness is sexy, in his eyes, for many reasons:

- Your clothes stick to you and he possibly gets to see a nipple outline.
- You look vulnerable because wetness is informal.

- He associates wetness with partially clothed or naked women (all men do – why else do they hang out at beaches and pools?).
- He imagines you in the shower.
- He imagines you in the shower together.
- His natural word association will leap from 'wet' to 'slippery' to 'sex.' That was difficult.

Introduce Him to your Lecherous Male Friends

A superb strategy because:

- It kickstarts his territorial mechanism.
- They're bound to be great guys which reflects well on you.
- He'll assume they all fancy you.
- It makes him realize he may have competition.
- It allows you to relax and show off a little.
- Male friends like to make their mark in front of new boyfriends and pull stunts like picking you up and flinging you over their shoulders.
- It gives you a legitimate excuse to show him he is not the be-all in your life.
- Your male friends can give you valuable insights into his behaviour (question: what does it mean when he didn't notice my new haircut? Answer: nothing at all).

Scare Note

If Mr Potential Right needs shaking up a little, one of your male friends should also be your ex-boyfriend. Of course, your Mr PR will be in two minds about this. First, he'll think you must be fairly stable (men, unless they are unhealthily insecure, do not go a bundle on you slagging off all your exes in a two hour rant). Second, he is a little freaked because he wonders if you still harbour feelings for this man. Third, he is jealous. He just is, unless he is totally sure of you. His reasoning: you have plenty of friends, why do you need the ex? He is history, so why is he present? Let him wonder — but not too much. Be affectionate to him in front of them — by which I mean hold hands — this will give him just enough reassurance, but not too much.

The Dinner Party of the Century

This is a devious way of showing him a great time without you having to be all-singing all dancing entertainment. It also demonstrates how popular and multi-talented you are, and lures him to your home. So:

- Invite your most entertaining friends.
- Cook your most reliable recipe and buy dessert from Marks & Spencer.
- Wear your slinkiest outfit.
- Add a twist to the dress code if you like – wigs, night-wear, school uniform.

Sexying Up Your Abode

In addition to the frilly knickers drying in the bathroom, there is many a home improvement ploy that will make him think you the foxiest creature he's ever come across in his life, bar an actual fox.

General Ambience

Clean, but not obsessively tidy. Even if he makes Stig of the Dump look like a manic obsessive, he will consider slobbiness gross in other people.

However, pristine tidiness terrifies most men – it makes them feel as if they've got to be on their best behaviour.

If you own the place, no doubt your impeccable taste will shine through however monstrous the legacy from the previous owner. Even if you haven't yet transformed the bathroom from its avocado/peat bog colour scheme to a white and chrome arrangement, don't flap. Only the worst sort of men judge you on an inherited bathroom.

Make sure you've aired the place so it smells nice and fresh when you come in. There's nothing worse than a flat that smells, however faintly, of cat wee. Especially if you don't own a cat.

Hallway

Answer machine – should be bleeping with at least six messages. Don't play them – say 'I'll listen to them later.' This is a double bluff: first, in case they are all from your mother who wants to be sure you did make an appointment for a smear test, second, what he doesn't know, hurts him – he wonders if the six messages are from six different men begging you to call them.

Kitchen

Fridge: possibly decorated with saucy fridge magnets – implies you have a sense of humour and aren't uptight. Doesn't have to be stocked brimful with food – a woman whose fridge contains one piece of mouldering cheese and green milk is endearing to most men. It suggests a soulmate. However – you probably can't lose because a bountiful fridge is equally impressive: first, if he's starving hungry it's very useful. Second, it is probably in pleasing contrast to his own bare fridge and suggests you are a woman of generous and sensual nature.

Notice board: crowded with flattering snaps of you surrounded by gorgeous men/glamorous girlfriends (not quite as photogenic as you in this particular instance) on holiday/at a party/having fun and looking gorgeous (gosh, you're so popular and beautiful). Far less vain than mounted, official photographs. Maybe a snap of you aged four? (If you were an odd-looking toddler forget it.) Also, invitations to this or that (gosh, you're so popular), the odd erotic playing card (nothing like a direct hit to the groin), postcards from exotic places (gosh, you're so popular), a scribbled note from your boss praising you for something or other (wow, successful too), memorabilia from a tacky gig (hey! what a fun gal!) – let your noticeboard be shorthand for the kind of person you want him to think you are (within reason – it should be you, airbrushed).

Lounge

Sofa: comfortable, squidgy, clean (no stains), useful if you want to snuggle up.

Bookcase: Let's be shameless. To give the impression that you're a well-rounded person, this should contain a pleasing variety of books, such as:

- Shakespeare, Jane Austen, Thomas Hardy, Charles Dickens, D H Lawrence (subtext: you're intelligent, you have depth and Lawrence is very sensual).
- Cult titles such as Jay McInerney, Elmore Leonard, James Ellroy.
- Frivolous books such as *Why Cats Paint*, and *Sex Lives of The US Presidents*.
- Anything on the supernatural to the girly – Jilly Cooper, Penny Vincenzi etc.
- Anything on design, fashion, or film stars.

It also helps if you've actually read them. Magazines also make a statement – possibly display a few copies of *Loaded* and *Esquire* (you're a fun woman, you like men). If you are in possession of *Bride And Homes* or similar, throw it in the bin before he arrives.

Music
As long as it isn't Elaine Paige anything goes.

Coffee Table
Maybe two wine-stained wine glasses are still residing there – we're not saying they denote a cosy evening in with another man, indeed they probably denote a cosy evening in with your sister, but our motto is 'let him wonder'...

Bedroom
Aha! If you've enticed him this far, unless you have a tarantula hunched on your pillow and your father standing in the corner, there's practically nothing in your bedroom that can put him off. Even so:

Bed
Preferably big, covered with a non-frilly, non-patterned duvet. If possible avoid checks. Alluring is a plain colour, usually white. I trust no woman needs to be told that a Scooby Doo duvet – while the dog in question is delightful – is not seductive. Boot out all cuddly toys – or pare them down to two – men hate them. If you've had Tedward since you were three weeks old, chances are he's looking raggedy and smelling worse – but because of his sentimental value

How to Seduce Your Dream Man

he's allowed. However, the hideous two-foot red poodle with googly eyes, bought for you three Christmasses ago by a tasteless ex, has no business in your bedroom or, for that matter, on earth. Ask yourself: is this poodle foxy? The kindest thing you can do is take Red Poodle to Oxfam – along with all his primary-coloured friends – and even then there's no guarantee they'll thank you.

Quick checklist:

- Hide any non-sexy bedwear, for example, tartan pyjamas, Marks & Spencer nightie.
- Put out on surreptitious show: 1 slinky pair of shoes, for example, pink fluffy mules, sparkly high heeled sandals.
- Hide all dirty clothes in laundry basket.
- Clear away all old coffee cups and other debris. All pizza crumbs should be vacuumed up.
- Minimize the number of china ornaments
- A few photos of mystery people, including at least one mystery man, should be tucked into the frame of your wall mirror. So what if they're all family? Good.
- Have candles, ready to light. Not scented ones – no need to over-egg the pudding.
- You can also buy floor lighting, very cheaply, from a good department store – superb for creating a romantic ambience, less obvious than candlelight – and anything's better than a vicious overhead glare.
- A vase of flowers – a bunch of yellow roses looks stylish and gorgeous and is usually available from your nearest

supermarket. However, if you've got the time to nip to a florist, they'll probably have a selection of exotic phallic looking blooms. Go for it.

All this is, of course, a mere addition to your unique taste – all quirky stuff is good – antique hat stand, football, tailor's dummy, dartboard – anything that surprises him in a non-unpleasant way. This is because a man enters a woman's bedroom for the first time in one of two ways:

- He doesn't notice the decor because you're too busy ripping each other's clothes off.
- He is a tiny bit self-conscious because nothing x-rated has yet occurred but is imminent, so he'll grab at any *faux* point of interest – 'Oh … a guitar … I didn't know you played … '

Wall decor – no teenagery posters. The must-have home accessory of the moment is a large abstract oil on canvas, painted by an artist friend of the family, worth more than the actual house, and given to you as a present.

How to Seduce Your Dream Man

STAGE 4:

Even Later

𝘟 𝘠 𝘠 𝘟 𝘐 𝘛 𝘠

You think the hardest work is over. Not so fast, sweetie. Grabbing his attention is the easy bit. Keeping it is harder, and this is the mistake many women (and men) make. Seduction should be continuous. Don't stop seducing him just because he is now officially your boyfriend, fiancé, husband – he is never a sure thing. Keep sight of what attracted him in the first place, keep doing it, and not only will he stay at heel, he'll become an absolute lap dog (while retaining, of course, his wonderful drive, wit, energy, independence, and charm etc., etc).

Never Use Threats, Veiled or Otherwise

Men are terrified that having a serious girlfriend signifies The End of Fun. So, just because you are teetering on the brink of a proper relationship, doesn't mean you can let all your insecurities hang loose. He is not going to give up his nights out with the boys, nor should you expect him to. So, if he announces he's going to a club with his pals, do the Tammy Wynette thing and button your lip. Not because you should stand by your man whatever happens, but because the most seductive thing you can do in a relationship is to let him have his own space. If you're worried he might snog someone else or worse, you have to face the fact that you have no power to stop him. Furthermore, it won't help to say anything warny-jokey-but-serious like 'Don't get off with anyone!' because:

- It sounds desperate.
- Stripped down to its raw material, it's begging.
- If he is the type of man who does get off with someone

when he's going out with someone else, you saying 'Don't' isn't going to dissuade him.

The most you can do is to:

- Make sure you're looking your ravishing best and if possible tempt him to bed a few hours before he leaves the house.
- Say 'Great, I was thinking of going out with Lisa and Tara that night.'
- Say something sweet and simple and caring but not grovelly such as 'Have a nice time, take care of yourself.'
- DON'T be tempted to add any provisos, for example, 'But not too nice!' or 'Ring me when you get back!' or 'Don't drink too much!' or 'Be good!' because his neck will tense and he'll think 'She is telling me what to do – I am no longer free.' Then he may panic, and – in a foolish attempt to convince himself that he is free – snog the first woman who wiggles past. Admittedly if he did, he would be an immature fool (*even immature fools know one of the basic prerequisites of entering a relationship is that you forgo certain freedoms, to take a random example: sleeping around*), but some men are outstandingly touchy, and the very immature ones can be easily goaded into an infidelity.

Trust Him

Tricky. If you don't trust him it is the hardest thing in the world not to question him, rifle through his pockets, spy on him when he goes out, check on him at the office, interrogate him when he comes home late ... okay, stop right there. This is not the behaviour of a seductress – it is the behaviour of a stalker. It is undignified, desperate and – if you are mistaken – it will drive him away. A good relationship is based on trust and if that is gone what is there? If you suspect he is cheating on you, keep your suspicions to yourself until you have proof way and above beyond reasonable doubt that he is playing away. Don't make sarcastic comments like – if, for instance, he comments on some two-timing footballer – 'and you should know.' Not only is it hostile, it's cowardly because it's an indirect form of attack. It will have no effect other than to make him defensive. Trust however – if he deserves it – makes him relax with you in the nicest possible way. It imparts a calm and unity to your relationship.

Quick Three: Sexy Games

- Truth or dare
- Strip Scrabble
- Monopoly*

---

* The loser gets so heated and huffy that the gloating winner has to kiss, tease, and tickle him/her into a better temper – and that can only be a good thing...

Don't Try to Force Intimacy

You spent the whole weekend together and it was blissful. You could be with him every moment of the day forever and ever and not tire of being together and you're sure he feels the same. Wrong and wrong! You want him to think you're an earthbound goddess but being omnipresent just won't swing it. He will find you far more wantable if you ration him. The temptation is to call just to say something cute, to make him fall in lust with you again, recount a funny thing that happened today to make him laugh and fancy you that little bit more ... Or, if you're driving back from seeing a friend, you *could* make a slight detour to his flat, even though you *said* you wouldn't see each other today but you know he'd be pleased to see you ... Resist! For seven reasons:

- He fancies you, okay? Relax. Give him time out to day-dream about you.
- Over-communicating is stifling, pressurizing, tensemaking. It means he'll stop seeing your presence as a treat.
- You constantly looming over him by phone or in person means he doesn't have to make an effort. If the

relationship is to be all you want it to be, it should be equal. You start acting the caretaker and he'll start acting like Little Lord Fauntleroy. Believe me – he won't need encouragement.

- His life won't stop dead just because he met you – nor should yours. Don't expect a 24-hour monopoly. If you do you'll frighten him.

- Maintain some space – no matter how much you want to be with each other, a degree of separateness is healthy. Especially if he is used to his singledom.

- True intimacy cannot be rushed, so don't force it. Talking and kissing till 5am is the most delicious soulmateyish feeling in the world – but hold back from asking him to move in with you. If – sorry to kill the mood here – an estate agent says 'You must exchange within two weeks or the deal's off' your natural suspicion is he's trying to stiff you. If there's no catch, there's no rush. Same goes with a relationship. If you try to cram 30 years of marriage-like intensity into the first three weeks he may back off.

- Even though most men are lazy, they like to chase. Correction – they love it. Don't offer yourself and your life up on a plate. Let him pursue.

Behave Like Brats

The reason most well-adjusted people like sugary food and doing frivolous things like feeding the ducks (although the ducks don't see it as frivolous) is because it reminds them of their childhood when – if they were lucky – they were safe, secure, unconditionally loved, and had fun. When you're a grown up – what with mortgages, earning a living, being scared into keeping fit – fun can be crowded out of your life. You fall into a routine. You never try anything new. You go to the same pub, the same restaurant, the same supermarket. But doing new and fun things together is a great way to bond. Making fools of yourselves together is intimacy-provoking. So, in the early days of your courtship – and the later ones if you have any sense – suggest:

- Going to feed the ducks.
- Playing on the arcades.
- Ten pin bowling.
- Sharing a knickerbocker glory.
- Paddling in the sea.*

* Will of course be foot-numbingly freezing, but cue lots of shrieking and girlish laughter – pedicure first so that even if they turn blue they're a fetching kinda blue.

- Going to the fair and eating candyfloss.
- Buying fish 'n' chips and eating them in the car.
- A trip to Toys R Us (purchase of play doh or water pistols compulsory).
- A game of football (frisbee if you must) in the park.
- Trying that glam new restaurant.
- Enrolling on a weekend surfing course together.
- Group visit to a karaoke bar.

Taking Up His Hobbies

Highly suspect, and best done in strict moderation. The goal is to impress him, and make him think 'Gee, we have so much in common – she loves Arsenal too.' Unfortunately, unless you really do love Arsenal too, this ploy can rebound on you and make you look like a sad loser with no personality of her own. If you think he'll be wowed by your knowledge of a sport/pursuit/subject that is traditionally favoured by men – there's no harm in swotting up a little, so that next time you are sitting with him and his friends you can drop a fabulous gem of specialist wisdom into the conversation. (You will have course have been tutored by an expert friend, or, you have been reading the sports pages for the past fortnight.) Then, leave it at that. You don't want to overdo it or he'll twig. One blast of unexpected genius he'll remember. Ten, and he'll start feeling threatened.

Real Life, Too Much

Mara, 28: 'I once had a crush on a guy called Chris. He supported Wimbledon. I so wanted to knock him down with my expertise on football, but I'd never even been to a match! I listened to all the sports news I could, taught myself about their home ground, their manager, how they were doing – all because I wanted Chris to fall for me. It didn't work. I'd engage him in conversation about football but I felt he knew what I was up to. He would grin patronizingly if I attempted to sound knowledgeable. In retrospect, I think if I'd been honest – football doesn't interest me at all – he would have respected me more. I don't think men are as impressed by ladettes as ladettes would like to think. It's too much like capitulation. Half the reason men like football is because they can all go off together and male bond. I don't think they like women trying to get in on that.'

Pursuing your own Hobbies

A much smarter ruse for about 38 squillion reasons:

■ Say your hobby is rollerblading (or boxing, pottery, or skydiving, as long as you have something you enjoy doing that doesn't depend on him calling you), you keep busy and entertained instead of moping around at home eating cereal straight out of the packet.

■ You are not always available – you are not always at home when he calls and, furthermore, your mobile is switched off. Therefore, he knows you have a life. He is frustrated – and, within moderation, frustration is the best thing ever for bringing Mr Right to heel. He wants a woman who has a life. The Mr Right sort of man has a terror of being trapped by a woman who doesn't have a life – whose sole source of entertainment is via him. Frankly it's a terrifying prospect for anyone. It is not flattering, it is a thought that will make him scarper. Most of us – men and women – loathe responsibility. Unfortunately it goes hand in hand with being grown up, and it entails tedious chores such as saving enough to pay the bills, sending birthday cards to cousins, getting that report into your boss on time and ensuring it kicks butt and not getting thanked for it. Responsibility is scary and yes, we know it has its rewards, but the idea of being responsible – worse, being responsible for someone else's happiness – is a petrifying thought.

Men don't want to think about things like that, and if they feel you need them in a too needy way their ardour may cool swiftly and without warning. Which is to say, do be unavailable – and tell him why too. Say 'I'd love to see you on Wednesday, but I have my skydiving lesson. Can we meet Thursday or Sunday instead?' (This way, you are being specific, giving him a clear choice of two possible days to meet rather than saying 'Can we do it some other time?' which is vague and leaves it up to him to suggest a precise day, something he probably won't want to do because effectively, he's been rejected once. Suggesting an exact alternative shows him you DO want to see him (positive feedback to balance the rebuff) and it also shows him that you are not so desperate for a man that you're prepared to cancel your whole life and rearrange it around him. Perfect.

He's Taking You for Granted

His mistake. But enough men make it. They get cocky and stop treating you with the degree of respect and lustfulness to which you are accustomed, for example, not returning calls on time, occasionally forgetting to turn up to meet you and your friends as planned, or flirting a little too heartily with other women...

For a start, you don't whine 'You're taking me for granted.' If you are brave – and peeved enough to take a risk – you say 'How would you feel if I saw other men?' That will shake him out of his complacency – and probably out of his chair too, as he leaps up and shouts 'What! No! I'd feel very upset and angry if you saw other men! Why do you say that?' To which you reply, 'You've seemed distracted recently, as if you didn't want an exclusive relationship.' Now, he is forced to be straight with you. Suddenly, you are not the grateful little woman, glad to scrape a pat on the head from her lord and master when he deigns to turn up. You are the powerful sexy woman he pursued because she was special ... and who doesn't suffer fools. Heel, darling.

If, however, you have been together for four years, the 'How would you feel if I saw other men' question might not go down a bundle. Instead, you mention 'a flattering thing' that happened today – a business client asked you out – out out! This will make him sit up. Then, a few days later, get your best friend to comment, *a propos* of nothing, how when you walked into a bar last week two gorgeous men asked to buy you (not her) a drink … it's as if they didn't notice the engagement ring … maybe it's because you're looking so slinky. He might not react immediately but all this information will be processed. He will be reminded that you are attractive to other men – even attracted to other men – and he knows how persuasive other men can be. He'll know, from what you've said, that you haven't strayed, but his complacency level will go into freefall. Good.

You make a big decision, excluding him. For instance, you say, 'I'm thinking of going on holiday, to the Greek Islands.' He says, 'But you know I don't like the Greek Islands.' You say, 'That's why you're not invited darling.' If this sounds simply too horrid and calculating, add innocently, 'Clare/Rachel/Laura is really keen to go. I thought we'd do a girls on tour. It'll be great.' If he is staring at you aghast, proceed with care. You do not want him to think you don't care about him because – as we know – this can lead a man to do silly things. So, say something neutral and friendly like, 'Shall we get a video out tonight?'

Then, whatever his reaction (probably a shrug) find an excuse to leave the room. The temptation is to hang around apologetically because you know you're manipulating him and feel nervous about his reaction. However, if you hover, you may be tempted to say something conciliatory. So move your ass. If – two hours later – you have got the video, ordered the pizza, and he's still acting huffy, blip off the video, shut the pizza box, and say 'What's wrong?' If he's got an ounce of prepossession he'll say sulkily 'Well, I didn't expect my girlfriend to go on holiday without me' (or some such piteous statement). You say, 'But darling, I thought you wanted some space ...' He is forced, whether he likes it or not, to clarify what he wants. Chances are, once he realizes you're only with him for as long as you want to be, he'll understand what he's got to lose, and that if he wants to keep it, he's got to try harder...

Quick One: Get Him Dancing

Lazy long term men are notorious in their determination to quit dancing. It's as if now they've found their dream woman, there is no reason to shake it about under flashing lights any more. Wrong! Dancing is sex standing up except more comfortable, it hustles all his feelgood hormones into action, and is bound to get him hot and bothered. It gives you the opportunity to jiggle and wiggle, rub up against him, and show off.

If you suspect that lazy long term man would laugh heartily and hurtfully at your dancing abilities, drag a friend to a salsa class – or similar – or hang out at a few clubs where no one cares what the hell you dance like, and practise. ('Darling, I'm going out tonight, with Sarah. No, not Pizza Hut, a club ... what? Because we want to dance. But darling, you don't like dancing ... ' Heh.)

It doesn't matter a bean what type of dancing you choose (not Morris dancing) – as long as it helps you to learn to move to the rhythm not against it. Then, when you feel you could give John Travolta a run for his money, force your man into a dancing situation. By this time, he'll be more open to persuasion. And, it doesn't have to be a hopelessly unrealistic 'Why don't we go ballroom dancing?' scenario. Just stick *Burning Love* on your lounge stereo and compete to perfect the Elvis swagger...

But What If You've Just Met Note

It's a good ruse if you've just met at a wedding, you've chatted all through dinner and the speeches, and everyone is set to boogey on down. At a wedding, asking a man to dance is not a massive deal – it's sharking under the guise of good wholesome family fun. If you are too feeble to pick on him specifically, suggest it to the table in general. If he's interested, he'll be hogging the dance floor before you can say Lady In Red.

Don't Ever Criticize his Mother

This makes grown men cry and hate you. (If he has a bad relationship with his parents, skip this one.) Men who get on well with their parents – not too dependent, not hostile – tend to be the most well-adjusted. Presuming he does adore them, to win his heart, you need to behave in a way that shows respect – not abject fear – and courtesy. Even if he is prone to letting his mother fuss around him, he will not appreciate it if you do the same. When you meet his parents for the first time – a big fat hairy deal, as we all know – he wants them to like you and you to like them. He will be acutely aware of how you interact with them.

How Not to Behave to Make him Melt

Even if his mother is about as warm as a deep-frozen Polar bear, don't snap back. This is not the time or place to make a stand. If you are bristly with indignation by the time you leave, bristle quietly. If the wealth of china ornaments ordered from Sunday supplements dominated the house – know it is not your place to pass judgement anywhere but in your head. If you do make a snide comment you'll learn

How to Seduce Your Dream Man

soon enough you said the wrong thing. Even if his mother makes Cruella de Vil look like that pink silvery sparkly fairy in *The Wizard of Oz* – button it. Most people – if they're lucky – grow up thinking their parents are perfect and the eventual realization that they're not is a profound shock. Many men retain a blind spot about their mother, and cannot bear to have any flaw commented on, especially by another woman (let's be brutal here) he barely knows. Unconditional adoration isn't the healthiest attitude, but it's by no means the worst. Indulge it. For now.

How to Behave to Make him Melt

Shake hands and make eye contact. When his parents offer you tea, jump up to help. Be courteous, not creepy – no need to morph into Pollyanna. Be chatty, not gobby. Be friendly, not too informal – no coy or cutesy references to the fact you're shagging their baby boy. Call them Mr and Mrs Blah until they say 'Oh call us Bill and Shirley!' If you can show sweet and genuine feeling towards his parents – or indeed his grandmother, or his favourite aunt – if he's a nice man, he'll love you for it. Most men have been spoiled rotten by an indulgent female relative and retain a soft spot for her. Kindness is an underrated seduction tool. It's a slow burner. Don't think that seduction is all about raw passion. If you want a one night stand it might be – but then again if you want a one night stand seduction is mainly down to the fact that you're there. Bringing Mr Right to heel for longer than five minutes requires deeper foundations. He sees you sympathizing with his Nan about her bad hip and offering to re-fill her teacup, and something in his heart flips over. Genuine sweetness is very beguiling.

Roll With It

(**NB** long term project)

Men are programmed to think that when a woman makes a request, then – on being ignored – repeats it, she is nagging. This is unfair. But that's how it is. They regard 'nagging' (and everything falls under its evil umbrella), from 'Did you water the plants?' to 'Your mother rang before and asked if you could call back' as something every man suffers from in a relationship. Men also regard 'nagging' as the most unsexy, unseductive thing in the world. Their faulty radar senses it in the most unlikely places. You need only say 'Can you pass the salt?' or 'Do you like this dress?' and they accuse you of nagging. They are hoping to intimidate you into silence and letting them run riot.

The smart woman – and I owe this wisdom to the psychiatrist Dr Raj Persaud – doesn't waste her breath. If her man wishes to leave his pants on the floor, forget to pay his credit card bills, starve his goldfish and so on, she lets him do so. She doesn't comment. She doesn't say 'Darling, please put your pants in the laundry basket.' Instead, she lets him experience the consequences of his inaction. She puts her laundry in the laundry basket and then she washes her whites. She leaves his stuff mouldering on the floor until the day he runs out of clean pants, and furthermore, runs out of recycled, turned inside-out pants, realizes that he is not rich enough to run out and buy new pants instead of washing the old pants, and — here's the punchline — clocks that maybe, if he had put his pants in the laundry basket and, moreover, washed them himself, he would not have to attend work wearing itchy bite-sized speedos under his trousers.

Fact: The washing machine works, he doesn't have to lug his underwear and a packet of Persil to the banks of the Thames, washing his pants isn't a hardship. He is hoist by his own lazy petard. The same goes for not paying his credit card bill. He is capable. If he asks 'Why didn't you remind me?' you say, 'I didn't want to nag you.' (Aside: Ha. Ha. HAH!) Let him receive a scary red letter then a threat of a court summons. Let him get a bad credit rating because he owes Amex seventeen pounds but can't be bothered to buy a stamp. An additional twist is to let him see the paradise that could have been — if only he'd had the foresight to pay Amex and wash his pants on time. You: 'I know! Why don't you visit your brother in New York next weekend on your Amex!' Him: 'I can't because I've got a bad credit rating and no clean pants … '

I hesitate to say the goldfish must die. Instead, move it to another tank in a secret location and let your man — at his leisure — spot that its habitual tank is empty. When he shrieks 'Where's Goldfinger?!' you say, 'Well, he was

How to Seduce Your Dream Man

floating at the top of his tank, so I buried him in the garden. I didn't want to upset you.' This way, you upset him mightily because he thinks Goldfinger has died of starvation and it is his fault. As he contemplates that it's anyone's right to report him to the RSPCA, say nothing at all. He'll think 'She lets me get away with murder. She doesn't nag, she doesn't say "I told you so." What a woman!' Keep Goldfinger hidden for another week while your man mourns his untimely passing.

Then, say 'I'm sure Goldfinger would want you to cherish another fish in honour of his memory.' At this point, he should nod miserably. Whereupon you, the kind, adorable, understanding woman that you are, triumphantly bring out Goldfinger – reincarnated during your witness protection programme as Fanta – in his new tank and present him to your man. If he notices a similarity, say 'I chose him specially.' If he persists in neglecting Fanta, go through the entire rigmarole again, including the digging of another small fish-grave at the bottom of the garden, but this time donate Fanta to your younger sister. He's learning the hard way to take responsibility for himself, yet when his friends gripe about being nagged he smiles smugly, a small glob of lust starts to throb, and he thinks 'Not my woman ... she's perfect.'

He doesn't know the half of it.

Never Stop Enjoying It

The mortgage, the phone bill, the electricity bill, the council tax, the gas bill, the car insurance, the car's MOT, the supermarket shop, the washing up, the office workload, the office politics, family traumas, stress, ill-health, exhaustion, arguments about who does what chores. Few of these tedious things impinge on a shiny new relationship because both parties are desperate to keep it as perky, fluffy, and fun-filled as a small puppy. Instinctively, you know what's seductive and what's not. Which is why on a first date you don't yap on for three hours about the misery of trying to move house or finding a decent rest home for your ill elderly great-aunt. You edit out what doesn't entertain and arouse.

Unfortunately, as the relationship progresses it often grows from a small puppy into a bad-tempered dog. Non-fluffy, rarely perky, and more snappy than fun-filled. Complacency engulfs you — he's seduced, at heel, you can relax. Not true. He's at heel — you don't have to attend as many dull parties, and there's a difference. As a wise relationship expert once said: A relationship is like a business. You have to put the work in. If people ran their work lives like they ran their love lives, they'd go bankrupt.

The moral is, keep fun a priority. Why bother bringing Mr Right to heel if the fun stops there? If that's the case you're better off single (and presume he'll think the same thing). Of course, a true Mr Right does not drop his leash and trot off just because you missed out on a day's fun but he is far more snuffly and jumpy-up (and likely to try and hump your leg) if you reward him for being Mr Right. The best sort of seductress never stops seducing her man for the duration of the relationship. She knows that seduction makes him feel wonderful, needed, appreciated, happy, sexy, and awed at being with such a fabulous woman.

We all need to be seduced – in the broadest sense. Appreciation – from our boss, our lover, our family – makes us try harder, it makes us feel the hard graft is worthwhile. If we don't get it, what's the point of trying? Traditionally, women are the ones who can't survive without frequent stroking and emotional feedback. Piffle. If anything, men need it more. So don't stint with Mr Right. Give generously. This doesn't mean your life together should be an act so never let him see you wearing sweatpants, and clear up his breakfast debris without whining. It means: your life together should be an adventure so ration the sweatpants wearing and get a cleaner. Don't take him for granted, ever. The following sound obvious, which is funny considering how easily they are neglected. So:

- Tell him you love him – say it like you mean it.
- Show him you love him – in more inventive ways.

- Be affectionate – kisses, full body hugs (arms and legs), bite his ear.
- Be unnecessarily kind – buy him his favourite after-shave, jam tarts, and excuse him from your grandma's birthday party because you know he'd prefer to be at the Metallica gig.
- If it doesn't matter profoundly, let it go – all men put duvet covers on duvets by actually getting inside the duvet cover and going from there.
- Play together – turn the washing up into a water fight, kick him under the table when your financially-aware friends divide up the bill precisely.
- Flirt with him – pinch his bottom as he walks up the stairs.
- Boast about him – to your friends, to his parents, to his friends, show him you're proud of him.
- Put a time limit on griping – about work/relatives/everything.
- Talk trivia – about why *The Hunt For Red October* makes you feel claustrophobic, why, if your cat wees in your underwear drawer, it's a protest not a sign of affection, about your childhoods and the naughtiest things you ever did – he killed the neighbour's budgie (he was trying to rescue it from the top of the curtain with the broom pole but crushed it instead), you forced your friend Amy to eat a caterpillar, about how, when you read a Jane Austen you start thinking like her characters, how he has found an internet page that instructs you on how to cheat at the N64 Goldeneye game.

How to Seduce Your Dream Man